DO YOU WANNABE A MODEL?

OR KNOW SOMEBODY WHO DOES?

Jeanne Frith & Tiffany Stanford

DEDICATION

We would like to dedicate this book to our wonderful mums, Beryl Chaudry and Lynda Frith. Without their support and help we wouldn't be where we are today.

Thank you both very much for all your love. xxx

2nd edition

© 2014 Jeanne Frith and Tiffany Stanford

Published by Jeanne Frith and Tiffany Stanford

The rights of Jeanne Frith and Tiffany Stanford to be identified as the authors of this work have been asserted by them in accordance with the Copyright, Designs and Patents Act of 1988.

All rights reserved; no part of this publication may be reproduced, stored in a retrieval system, or transmitted in any form or by any means, electronic, mechanical, photocopying, recording or otherwise without the prior written consent of the publisher or a licence permitting copying in the UK issued by the Copyright Licensing Agency Ltd, www.cla.co.uk

ISBN 978-1-78222-295-8

Book design, layout and production management by Into Print
www.intoprint.net
+44 (0)1604 832149

Printed and bound in UK and USA by Lightning Source

Contents

Introduction 5
Jeanne's Introduction 7
Tiffany's Introduction 11
Wannabe Workshops Success Stories 15
Model Agencies 17
Types of Modelling 19
How to Join an Agency 24
What is a CV? 25
Your Modelling Career 25
Photography Work 26
10 Tips on Posing in front of the Camera 30
A Look Book 31
Fashion Shows 31
A Running Order 36
Promotion and Exhibition Work 37
Exhibition and Stand Modelling 39
Part Modelling 40
Fittings 41
Glamour Modelling 43
What is a Showreel? 45
Video, Presenting TV and Commercials 45
Castings 46
Go-Sees 47
Accepting Rejection 48
Testing with a Photographer 49
Contact Sheets 51
Portfolios 53
Mini Book 56
A Disc 56
Composite Card 57
Model Bag 58
Direct Booking 59
A Model Release Form 60

Invoices	60
Dos and Don'ts of Modelling	61
Modelling Scams	62
Stylist/Styling	63
Specialised Underwear	66
Hairdressing	68
Skin Throughout the Years	73
Skin Types	78
Cleansing, Toning and Moisturising	79
Anti-Ageing Products	81
Face Types	81
How to Apply Make-up to Ethnic Skin Tone	83
Nine Steps to Natural Make-up for a Casting and Day Make-up	84
Make-up Tips for Mature Skin	85
Evening Make-up	87
Eyes	88
Lips	90
Applying False Tan	91
Body Brushing	92
Make-up Brushes	92
Eyebrows	95
How to Look After Your Nails	96
Healthy Diet	100
Exercise	101
Contacts	104
Beauty Competitions	104
Example Invoice	108
Glossary	108
Jeanne's Funny Modelling Stories	110
Tiffany's Funny Modelling Stories	112
Jeanne's Modelling Diary	116
Tiffany's Modelling Diary	120
Our Final Words	123

Note: all prices correct at time of going to press.

INTRODUCTION

Jeanne and Tiffany established Wannabe Workshops in 2009. Tiffany approached Jeanne to start holding model workshops and Jeanne had always wanted do something like this as she had always felt there was a gap in the market for young potential models. When Jeanne and Tiffany started modelling, the only help available was in the form of the Yellow Pages which gave agencies' telephone numbers and addresses. There were many unanswered questions for them both: who do you approach? Where is the best place to start? Today, many people search the Internet as soon as they want help finding information. There is plenty of advice out there at your fingertips, many of it sound and useful, however the Internet is unregulated and ANYONE can set up a website. Now the questions are: Is this reliable? Is this agency legitimate? Can I trust these people? You will read and hear about many companies that claim to be agencies but will gladly take your hard-earned money for photo shoots, prints and advice that is not useful! Now there is Wannabe Workshops for everyone who wants to be a model and needs a helping hand to get started!

During the start of our modelling careers our supportive parents wasted huge amounts of money (which neither of them had!). We both spent unnecessary money on photographers that took great pictures for the family

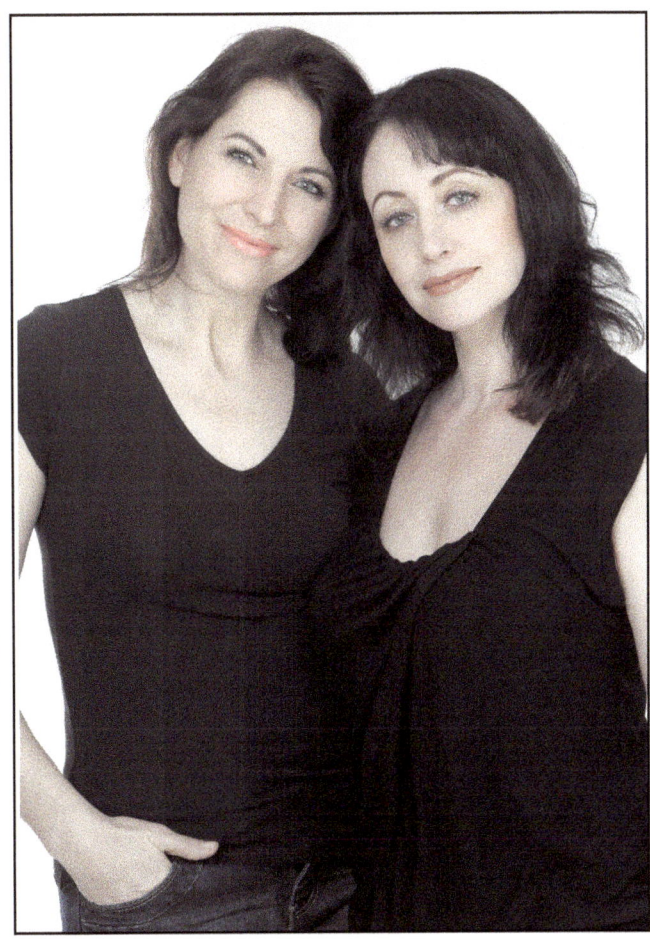

Jeanne and Tiffany 2012.

album but totally inappropriate photographs for the cutting edge of fashion, which were what the agencies were looking for! The photographers we worked with were great people but just didn't have the experience we needed to get a good portfolio, resulting in us paying out for numerous unsuitable prints. We didn't have anyone to teach us how to pose in front of the camera, how to 'sell' a product by modelling it, or how to be natural in front of strangers. We had to teach ourselves these things and it took a long time to learn! If someone with experience had taught us how to model like teachers teach us maths at school, we would have learnt so much faster and saved a lot of money. Basically, we are providing what we craved for when we started modelling. We do not promise that if you attend our workshops, or read our book, that you will have a glittering modelling career. However, we passionately believe that by taking our advice and following our tips and rules, you will achieve your full potential a lot quicker and spend a lot less money on your route to success! We teach you all the basics of modelling – all about the industry, what to do and what not to do, creating an eye-catching portfolio, hair and make-up for photography and much more! Jeanne (our photographer) knows exactly how you probably feel in front of the camera for the first few times, and teaches you how to move and feel confident in front of the lens.

We will be honest about everything and it goes without saying, like with many jobs, that you will have to spend some money to set yourself up. But we will make sure you do not waste your money and only spend what is absolutely necessary to begin your modelling career.

We believe that, with 40 years of modelling experience and completion of various academic courses between us, we are qualified to help you on the road to a fulfilling career in this field. Our experience is invaluable and we aim to nurture everyone who attends our workshops and reads our book into becoming the best model they can be. We are prime examples of the fantastic opportunities that modelling can offer. This fabulous career can be exciting, you can be your own boss, pick and choose what jobs you want, travel and meet some amazing people on the way. Each day can offer variety, and it can be a lucrative career if you work hard. Modelling can open many doors to other possibilities like presenting, photography, fashion designing... the list is endless and with our help you can get a head start!

JEANNE FRITH

I was born on the 27th October 1970 in Mortimer near Reading. I am the second eldest of four girls of Lynda and Ian Frith. We moved to the Midlands when I was four. I remember writing to local model agencies at the age of 13 wanting to be a model and asking them for advice and whether they would take me on their books. I wasn't conventional model material, being very gangly and not particularly striking looking. I wasn't photogenic and looked very plain in pictures.

When I was 15 my sister won a local beauty competition, *Miss Stourport*. Sarah hadn't shown any interest in modelling and had entered it when our mum spotted an advert in a local newspaper. A photographer from a local newspaper came to take some pictures of Sarah and I was the official leaf thrower! I remember saying to the photographer, "You will be taking pictures of me next year when I win!". This was totally out of character for me because I was never that confident, but sure enough the following year the same photographer turned up to take pictures of the new *Miss Kidderminster,* which was me. It was my first beauty competition and it was fantastic. I loved every minute of it and not just because I won. I loved the whole experience and at one point I was so busy staring at the contestants my Mum said "Jeanne aren't you even going to brush your hair?".

I entered competitions regularly and won a few. I won *Miss Photographic* in 1988, securing me a place in the last televised showing of *Miss UK*. I didn't win or get placed but it was a brilliant experience. I went on to win a few more and the most memorable ones were *Miss Birmingham*, where my dad heard one of the other fathers say "You call that beauty?" when my name was read out as the winner; *Miss BRMB* as it was my mum's birthday and held at the NEC and I don't know if they did but it felt like the whole audience stood up when I won! And *Miss Merry Hill* as my then boyfriend, now husband Ross, had come to support me.

At this stage in my career I was getting a fair amount of modelling work. I had started off doing promotions but was having to turn down better paid jobs, so in the end I stopped doing promotions. This was a risk as promotions were more reliable, but luckily my decision paid off!

I went to Milan to work for three months when I was 22, and this was a great experience: living with a load of girls from all around the world, going to castings everyday. I did some fantastic testing too. In fact the first test I did was the first morning I arrived at the agency. They had got my shoe size down wrong, thinking I was American. It was only at the end of the shoot that I realised I had been squeezing my size 7s into size 5s! The eye make-up was very strong and the lip liner went right over my lips. When we finished, the agency gave me a list of castings and go-sees. I asked about my make-up. "Just take off your lips the eyes will be ok." It was February and during the afternoon it snowed. I wasn't keen on taking the trams and buses so I kept to the underground and walked. By the time I got to the last casting of the day the client looked at my book and said, "You have something on your face, I think you should go to the bathroom." I had black eyeshadow and mascara all over my face! I didn't get any jobs from those castings or go-sees!

Throughout my teens I completed my Duke of Edinburgh Award and went to London to collect my Gold from Prince Philip. I took my mum and she loved it. What a great experience the whole occasion was, from camping for one night to ending up touring the English countryside, camping for four nights and covering 30 plus miles. My final study was on old church buildings, drawing them and collecting literature. The Duke of Edinburgh Award was a great thing to do and I would recommend it to anyone.

Like Tiffany, I also joined a band. We were called The Electric Energy People's Boogie Revolution Band !!!! We did have some amazing talent in our band but sadly it wasn't me or my gorgeous best friend at the time, Tiffany (not the same Tiffany). The lead singer, Lee, was fantastic and really did have talent. We did a demo tape and went to London to try and get signed up. It was just like that advert, although he didn't say we would go a long way!!! Shame, as when we did our one and only gig, I loved it, but I can't sing at all. In the end I got sacked when I went off to Milan.

When I was pregnant with my daughter I didn't want to waste a year by not working so I went to college and did a theatrical and media make-up course. After the year I went back and did fashion and photographic. Then my mum asked if I would go with her on a photography course. I wasn't into it but I went with her anyway. We stayed on for two years and funnily enough I now earn more money through photography than I do through modelling.

Top: Modelling test aged 16. In the Electric Energy People's Boogie Revolution Band. Second row: Collecting my Duke of Edinburgh Award. Winning Miss Superstore. Third row: Wedding day. Mum and the blushing bride. As a baby 10 months. Aged 7, so cute. Bottom: My wedding to Ross in 1996. With my sisters at my elder sister's second wedding – Helen, Linsey, Sarah, Jeanne.

Jeanne's Introduction

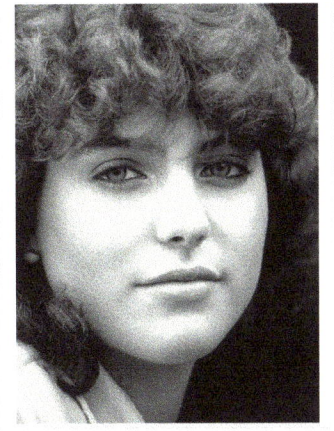
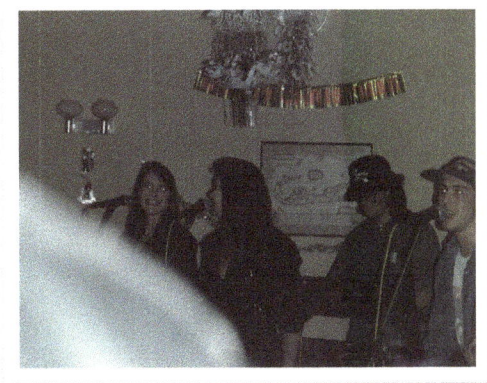
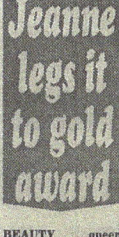
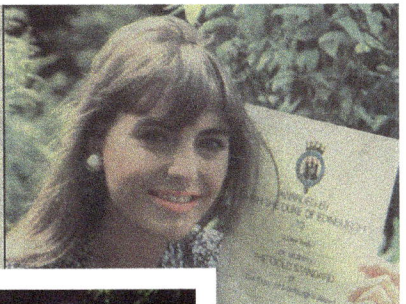
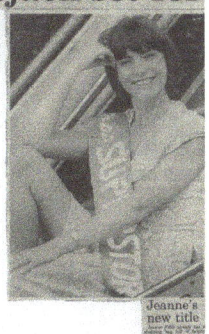
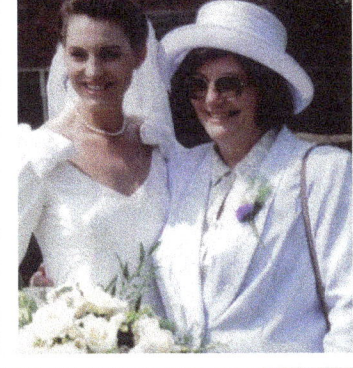
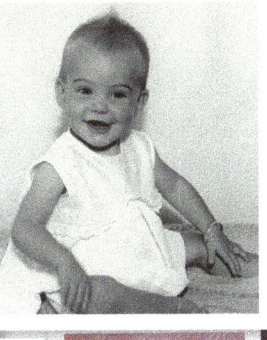
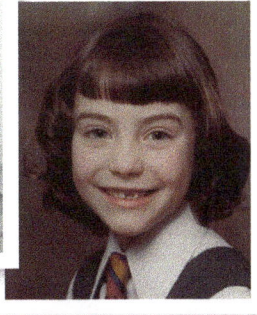
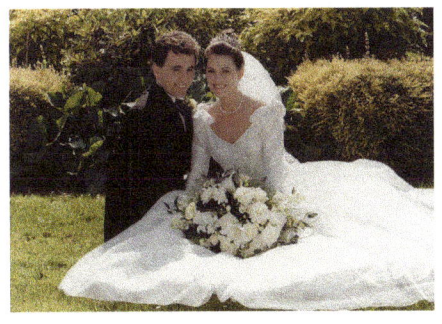
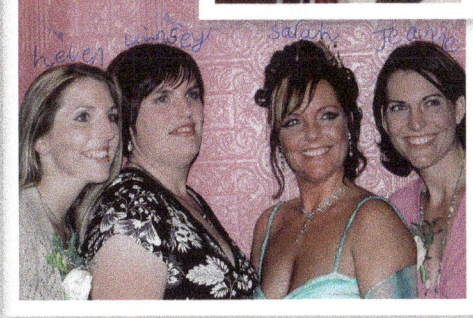

Do You Wannabe a Model?

My mum, whom I loved dearly and who I was very close to, had a brain haemorrhage when she was 54 and died very suddenly. This was a very difficult time for me and I miss her every day. Without my mum and her support and encouragement I would not be where I am today. I would not be the woman I am today. She brought out the best in me and was so proud of my modelling career.

I have done 1,000s of jobs for numerous brands over my modelling career. I have taken part in either fashion shows, photoshoots or videos for the following companies: Porsche, Kelloggs, Sunseekers, Pretty Polly, Littlewoods, Cashmere Centre, Marks and Spencers, Avon, J D Williams, John Lewis, Clarks and Jean Paul Gaultier, to name a few.

I came across Arbonne as we wanted to recommend a fabulous product to our Wannabe clients. I wanted to feel comfortable using a product that was safe, pure and beneficial. Arbonne is all of these. We sell products from Babies to Anti ageing and everything in between. I love the products so much that I am an active independent consultant and I am building a huge team teaching them how to turn an everyday expense into a residential income. To learn more about these award winning products, to place an order or to learn about the amazing business opportunities, go to http://jeannefrith.myarbonne.co.uk

I am married now and have two beautiful children. I am nowhere near as busy with modelling as I used to be, but still model today. It's such a diverse and interesting industry. Why would I give it up?

Lots of luck

Jeanne Frith x

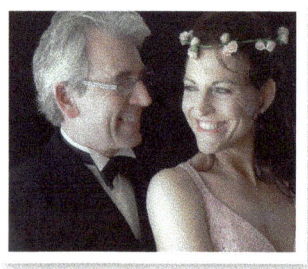
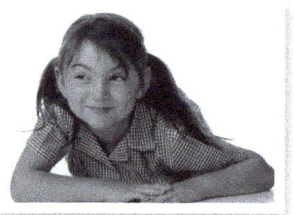
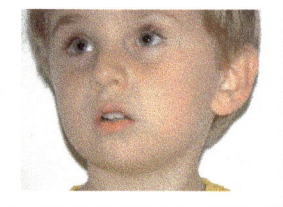

With Ross at the Winterfold ball 2011. Midsummer Night Dream theme. My daughter Taylor aged 5. My son Carter aged 3.

TIFFANY STANFORD

I was born on the 31st December 1969 in Birmingham. My wonderful mother Beryl was a single parent and surrounded me with a huge amount of love and protection. I had a wonderful childhood with many fond memories, mainly of spending every moment I possibly could with my two ponies Star and Goldie, going to lots of horse shows which I loved competing in and winning rosettes at, the ponies were my life. Straight from leaving school at 16 I learnt the trade of hairdressing and beauty and ran one of my mother's hair salons. After entering *Miss West Midlands* 1988 (my first beauty competition) I then joined a Birmingham agency called Number One and started part-time modelling until I was 21. I then did full-time modelling and promotional work until I was 25. During my successful modelling career I did a wide variety of modelling jobs including photographic, TV work, part modelling, tours, catwalk, exhibition shows, fittings, lingerie/tights modelling and magazine work. Some clients I have worked for are Vivienne Westwood, Umberto Giannini, Charnos, Speedo, Trevor Sorbie and Pretty Polly. I have appeared in many magazines, e.g. *OK*, *Chat*, *Take a Break*, *Hello*, and various wedding and hair magazines. I have also put a showreel together and have done some presenting work for various companies. I have had a very busy fulfilled career and have enjoyed my experience very much. I loved the friendships I made, the travelling, staying in beautiful hotels and generally having good fun. During my career I was lucky enough to have

11 months old. With my pony Goldie at a show winning loads of rosettes and a cup for best rider. Bottom: with pony Star. Right: at Hawkesley school 1977 – I look like a boy with this haircut.

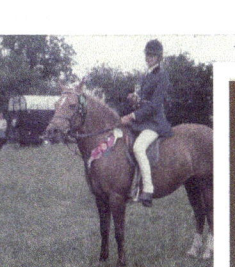
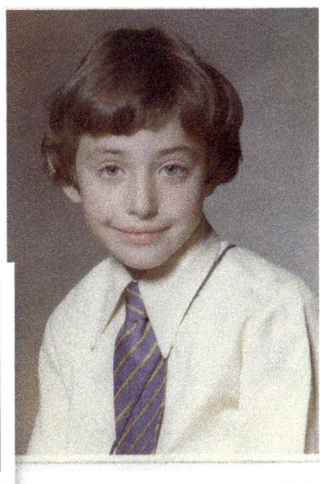
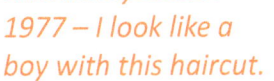
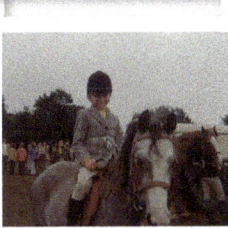

met and worked with a lot of celebrities: Boy George, Sir Bob Geldolf, Kylie Minogue, Victoria Beckham and Caprice, to name a few. I enjoyed the many extra advantages of being a model but my favourite was going to a lot of film premieres; one was attending the film premiere of *A Perfect Storm,* at which I was standing right next to the gorgeous George Clooney! Whilst modelling on a Trevor Sorbie tour I and four other model friends created a model girl band called *Barefaced Chic* (it was all about how we looked and that we were models). We had a manager, did some recording in a studio in Kingsley and Birmingham, and had some gigs lined up. We could have been *Girls Aloud*

Top: In model band Barefaced Chic (I'm second from right). With my pals wearing my designs from university, partying in Sheffield. Bottom: first photo shoot at 16, in Northfield by Stanley Dolphin Photography – they even put my picture in their window. What's with wearing all the gold? Middle: Getting my BA (Hons) in Fashion Design. Right: University degree publicity card for final collection.

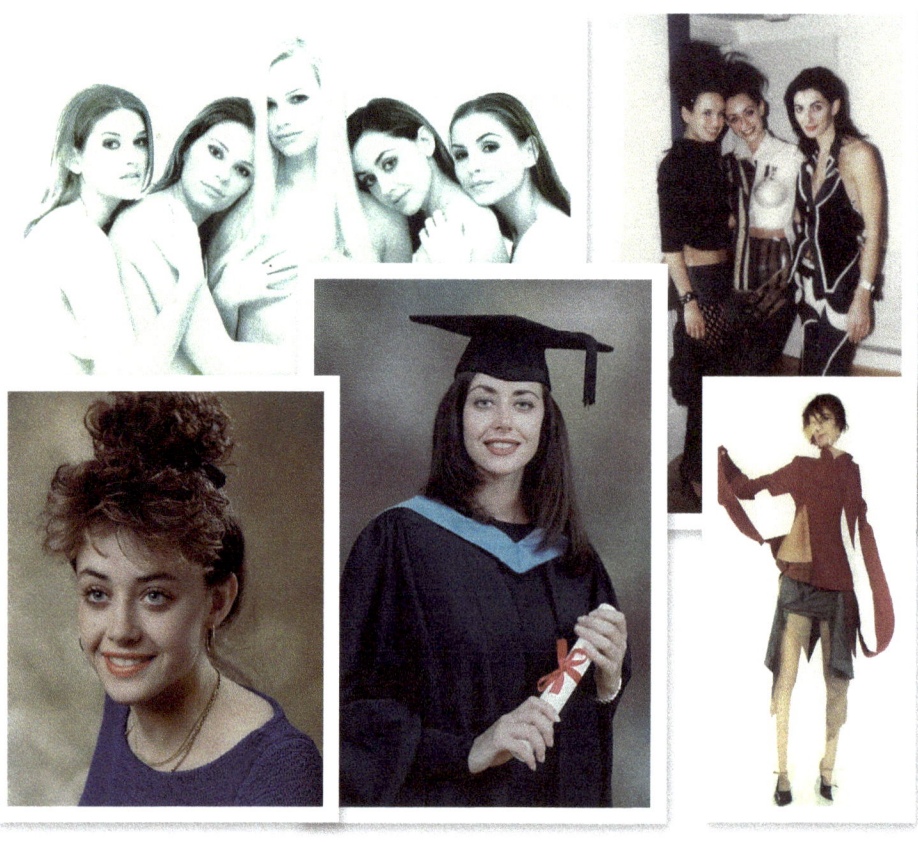

TIFFANY'S INTRODUCTION

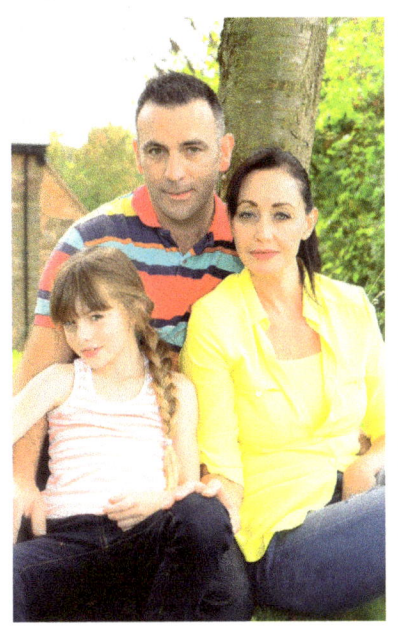

Family photograph taken in Ledbury by Jeanne Frith. My gorgeous husband Tim and beautiful daughter Tia - 2014.

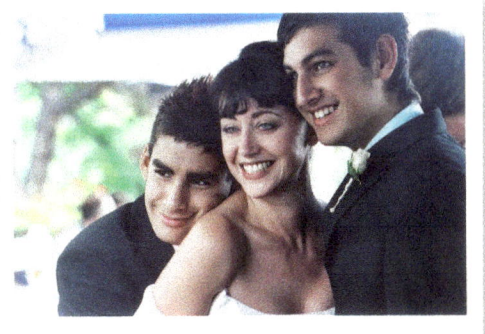

The best day ever, getting married in Prague to Tim (where he proposed three years earlier) on 1st September 2006. I'm with my brothers Karim (left) and Zia (right).

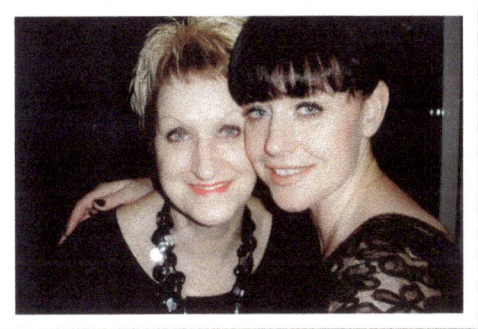

Tiffany (39) and mum (59), New Year's Eve.

if we could have actually sung well and had some real talent!! Hilarious but fun! During my career I also won various beauty competitions: *Face of the Midlands* 1988, *Miss Beautiful Eyes* 1991 and *Miss Great Britain* in 1992. I also represented my country in the American *Miss Universe Pageant* held in Thailand. For a month, all of the 78 contestants from around the world were treated like celebrities, meeting the King and Queen of Thailand, attending lots of organised visits and signing lots of autographs!

During my beauty competition days I was asked to open many different shops and give out awards to various competition winners around the UK.

At 25 I decided to go to university for four years, where I achieved an HND and BA Hons Degree in Fashion Design. I feel that this is the best and bravest thing I have achieved during my career: to go back into studying as a mature student and miss out on some great modelling jobs, one of which was the casting to appear in the Stanley Kubrick film *Eyes Wide Shut*. A few of my friends appeared in the nude masked scenes. I excelled in the fashion course and won various competitions during my studies at Northampton University.

I am now an award-winning fashion designer and have sold my designs in Top Shop London and in outlets around the UK. Having been on the judging panel of *Miss Great Britain* in 1998 (when I sat next to Simon Cowell – yes this is before he was famous!), I was asked to design the Miss Great Britain 1998 national costume for the *Miss Universe Pageant*, which was a great honour and received publicity on the *This Morning* TV show. I currently run a successful promotion and corporate clothing design and manufacturing business and have been a winner of the *Small Business of the Year* award – www.barebackfashion.com

Clients include: Imperial Tobacco, Captain Morgan, WKD, Arsenal Football Club and Fiat. I am a fully trained and qualified image consultant. For further information, look at www.tiffanystanfordimageconsultant.com. I have also been a fashion stylist for many different magazines, music shoots and catwalk shows.

I have taught fashion to both young and mature people at schools and universities as a visiting lecturer, which I enjoy hugely as it is important to me to give support to the up-and-coming youth of today.

I have been involved in the creative fashion industry all my working life and feel very lucky to have, during my career, achieved everything that I have, and I am grateful to have gained so many years experience. I am very passionate about *Wannabe Workshops*, which I had the idea to set up in 2009, and enjoy giving all my knowledge and experience (which I feel is priceless) to up-and-coming models of today during the workshops.

I hope you enjoy our book!

Tiffany Stanford. x

WANNABE WORKSHOPS SUCCESS STORIES

"Hello, I'm Isabella Rowles. I attended Wannabe Workshops 2 years ago, since then I have had a lot of success with my modelling career, I have joined a variety of agencies, including Alan Sharman, Elliott brown, DNA and Source. At the workshop I was given a list of reputable agencies to contact, which I am now signed with. My pictures for my start up portfolio were taken at the workshop along with having my hair and make up professionally done, with these pictures I used them to send to the agencies and as a result, it kick started off my modelling career. I was taught a lot about the dos and don'ts of the industry, and was given a lot of advise to help me with my career. Along with all of this, I was even taught how to catwalk. The day gave me invaluable advise and the confidence to reach out into the modelling world. For this I am very thankful, as without the information given mistakes could have been made, for example approaching dodgy agencies. Overall, the workshop was a fantastic and unforgettable experience in which I thoroughly enjoyed."

"My daughter Kelly has always been a star in my eyes but lacked confidence. Kelly attended Wannabe Workshops modelling day and wow what a transformation. She now stands up with a new found confidence and glow. On the day she learnt how to pose, catwalk, found out about modelling secrets, the dos and don'ts of the modelling industry. Kelly also went away with some show stopping portfolio pictures to help further her modelling career. I would highly recommend the workshop to all budding models and pageant girls." – Tracey Cook

"Charlie Matthews, after winning our Facebook competition, recently attended our Workshop. She thoroughly enjoyed the day and left with yet more confidence and self belief. Charlie is such an inspiration to everybody and is an amazing, brave little girl. She is achieving great things, is winning lots of beauty pageants and has recently appeared in Bella magazine sharing her story. Although it is sad, she doesn't let her autism or other disabilities, which she deals with on a daily basis, stop her from doing anything." – Jeanne and Tiffany.

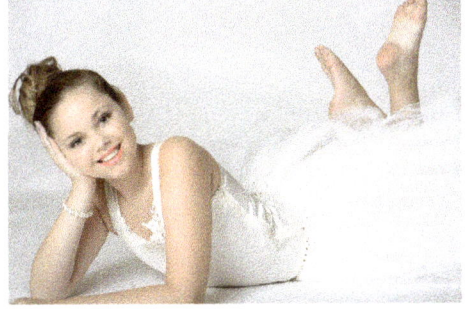

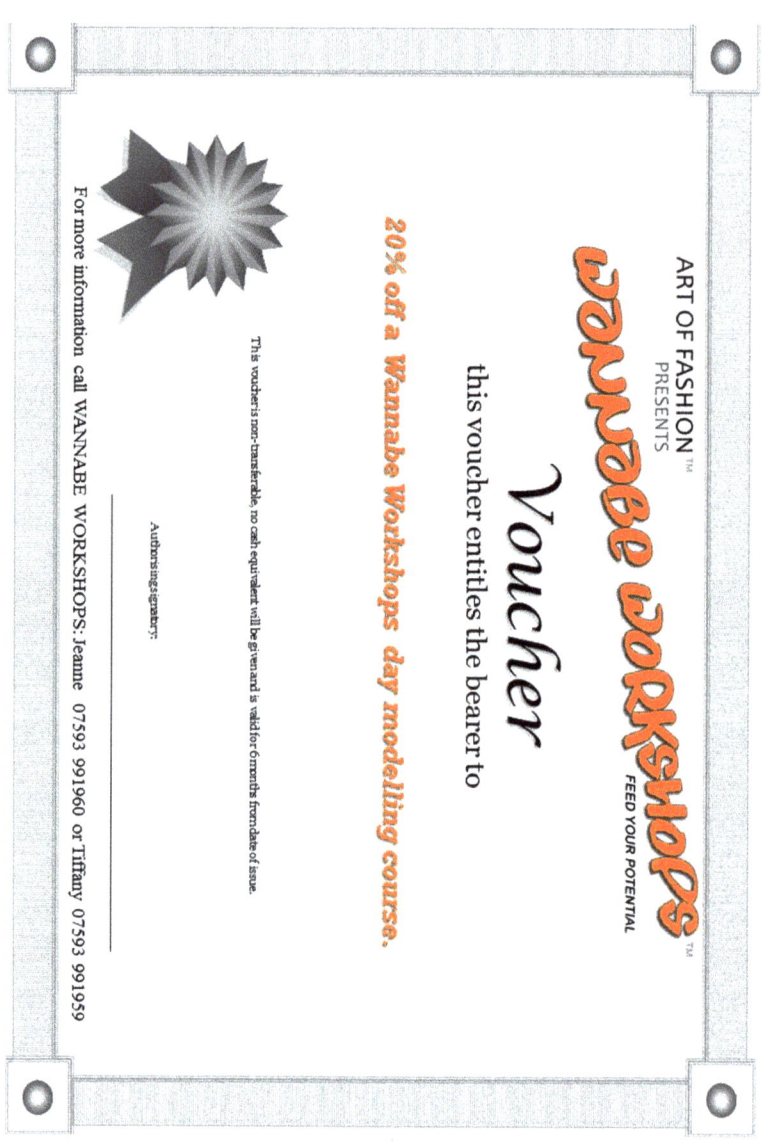

Call Wannabe Workshops on: 0800 170 1960

MODEL AGENCIES

A model agency is a business set up to find models all different aspects of work. There are lots of different types of model agencies which represent specific people and ages, e.g children agencies, real people, character models, plus size models. Make sure you are with the right agency to suit you. It will be their job to get you different types of work, sort out the fees and collect the monies for you, and in return you pay them a commission. This varies in different towns, but on average the commission is between 20%-30% of your total fee. When you get your first job, it's important to understand clearly what you are going to come out with. If you are not sure, make sure to ask.

It is best to seek representation by one agency per area. Model agencies do not like you to be with any others in the area. However you can join different agencies in different areas e.g. you could be represented by three different agencies: one in London, one in Birmingham and one in Manchester without a problem. You can, however, be represented by as many promotion agencies as you want. If you are taken on by one of the main agencies in London, then they may require you to be exclusive, as they will be known as your 'Mother Agent'.

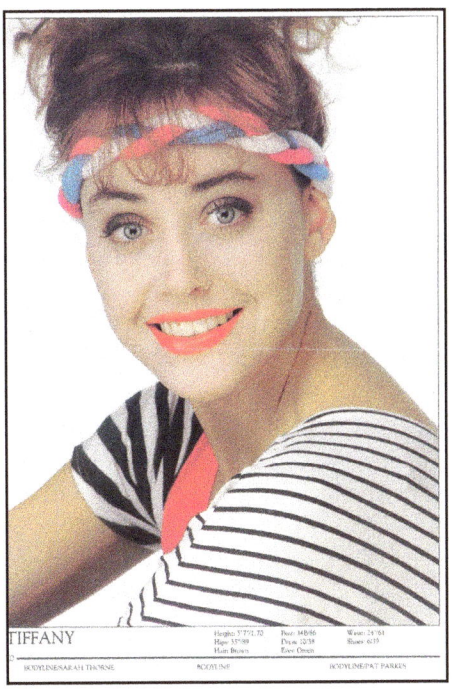

Tiffany's favourite agency model book shot. Olivia Newton John eat your heart out. In Pat Parkes/ Bodyline model book. Model books are not in use any more as most clients look on an agency's website.

If you have the potential it is very easy to join an agency. We would advise finding local agencies and sending in a head and shoulder shot plus a full length picture (a clear digital shot or snap shot is ok to use) together with all your details attached i.e. height, dress size, shoe size, hair and eye colour, and await a reply. In most cases they will respond even if it's a "no". You could call them and ask them if they have an open day, but this is mainly in London. The big agencies tend to have an open morning from 10am-12pm where anyone can just drop in. We would recommend that you telephone and ask for a meeting. At some stage, even if you have sent in pictures, they will call you up to arrange an interview where you will have to go and see them. This way they can just check that you haven't got a wart on the end of your nose that has been airbrushed out of all your pictures and check your sizes etc!

When you go for your interview keep clothes simple and make-up to a minimum, so that the agency can see your skin and bone structure clearly.

You should NEVER pay a fee to *join* an agency – the legislation was enacted in 1998 – although it is normal to pay for any testing that the agency organises, or indeed if your photograph goes in their model book (if they have one). Payment is also normal if you are on their website, or if you have a composite card made through the agency. (Comp cards are not really used that much these days but it's good to leave one at any castings that you go to.)

Most agencies take an average of three months to pay. When you do get paid, you will not have paid any tax or National Insurance if it was photographic or fashion show work. It is your responsibility as the model (if aged 16 and above) to sort out and pay tax and National Insurance yourself. If you don't understand about tax and National Insurance, you could pay an accountant, which we highly recommend doing. They charge on average of between £200-£500 and will work out your annual finances. In the end they will save you money, but if you have any questions or don't want to use an accountant your local tax office is always happy to help you. Remember to keep all your receipts for petrol, clothing as you can deduct all of these expenses from your year end tax bill.

Promotional agencies normally pay within six weeks. You do, however, have to pay tax and National Insurance at source and the agency will take it off your money. If at the end of the year you have paid too much tax, you will get a rebate.

Try and save at least 25% of any money that you earn. At the end of your tax year (most run from April-March) you will have some towards your tax bill and some savings left over if the bill is less than you've saved!

TOP TIP

Never give a client your own personal details to cut out the agency. Most agencies will find out if you do this. They will not trust you to represent them again and although you may get direct work from one client, you risk losing any future work from the agency. In the long run it is not worth it!

TYPES OF MODELLING

If you want to be a model but are unsure which agency is right for you, you first need to understand which market you fit into, as there are many different modelling agencies around. Many agencies specialise and represent a certain type of model while other agencies will represent all different ages, shapes, sizes and heights. It is possible you could enjoy a modelling career from birth right through to old age. Below are some modelling examples:

Child modelling – Modelling can be a great way to boost your child's confidence, get some fun experience and earn some good money, but a parent will need to be flexible and be able to put a lot of time into their child's career too, as they will need to be their chaperone. Child modelling can start from birth, through the toddler years and continue up to 16 years old. There are a lot of agencies who will just specialise in these age groups. You can expect to get various modelling jobs from photographic work to fashion shows, promoting lots of different products, such as toys and clothing.

Your child's personality and attitude are key to any child modelling. Children need to be easy to work with and direct, be patient and be at ease with strangers. NO temper tantrums or sulking will be tolerated!

Fortunately there are strict laws in place for child modelling to ensure that children are not exploited and don't miss out on education. Licences are required from the local council to permit any child under 16 to work and to decide on the number of hours. It is vital that a child's education always comes first.

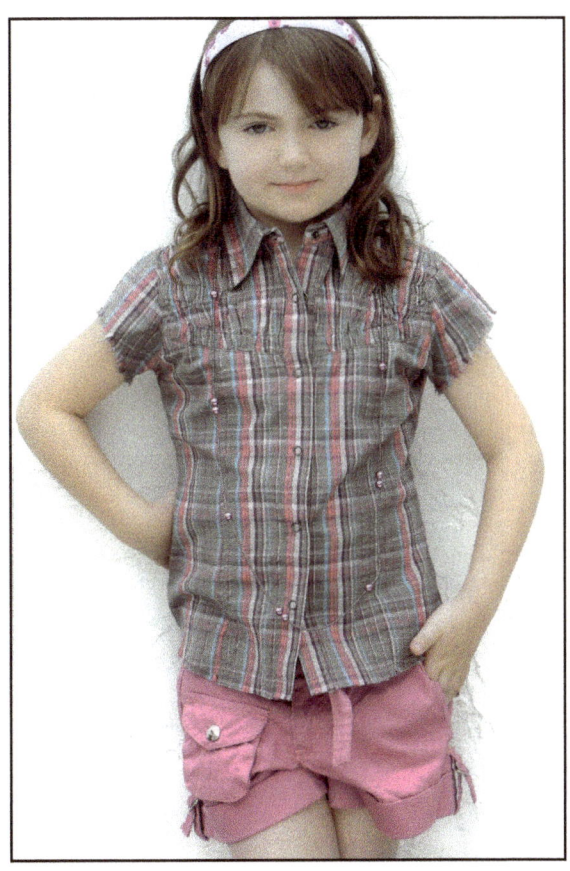

Taylor aged 7. Courtesy of Model Camp photography.

Do You Wannabe a Model?

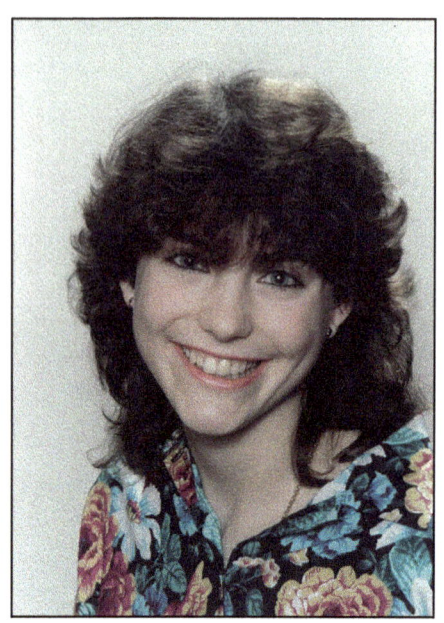

Jeanne's first photo shoot, aged 16. It was advertised in the paper, cost £50 but resulted in no work.

Teenage modelling – As a teenage model, you will be aged from 13 upwards and you can expect to get pretty much all the same types of modelling work as adults. The requirements are the same as general modelling i.e. beautiful facial features, a good personality and good body proportions. Again your parent will be required to be with you and be your chaperone. Your education should always come first!

Petite modelling – If you are particularly small in height and size – anything under 5 feet 5 inches tall – you could work as a petite model. You may not ever be a catwalk fashion model, but there are lots of other areas of work you can expect to get, for example fitting work, part modelling, beauty work and promotional work. You might even get away with doing some younger teenage modelling but get an adult's rate of pay.

Tall modelling – If you are 5 feet 10 or taller you will be welcome at most general agencies, you could easily be a catwalk fashion model, but also expect to do fitting work as it is a growing trend for taller available fashion brands.

Unique modelling – This is a niche market and really specialises in people who may have specialised features or unusual quirks that may make an advert stand out. We are all unique individuals so embrace who you are. The work that you can expect to get will be exactly the same as all the other modelling areas, such as photographic jobs, part modelling and TV commercials. A great agency to be with is www.ugly.org

Pregnant modelling – At some stage you may be pregnant. During a pregnancy a woman blooms, skin and hair shine and she generally looks radiant. Why not show yourself off and model throughout all the different stages of pregnancy? You may also want to continue to model with your newborn or as part of a family.

Types of Modelling

You will need to be photogenic and be in proportion, and you can expect to get various photographic jobs modelling clothing and baby products etc.

Plus size modelling – If you are a size 14 upwards, embrace your curves ladies, and let's not forget the larger men, and be a plus size model. As long as your body is in proportion you can get work. The fashion industry is finally realising that fashion is for all shapes and sizes and that the average sized woman in the UK is in fact a size 14. You will be required to do fittings, fashion shows and photographic work.

Fitness modelling – Fitness/athletic models specialise in body work as they have great figures. This can be aimed at either women or men. They also may have a specific speciality at some sport, e.g. diving, rugby or boxing. Other agencies may get the occasional job that fits these requirements but the best agency is www.wathletic.com which is based in London.

Family modelling – This is basically a fictitious family (most ages welcome) usually consisting of a mum and dad, and a brother and sister. It is required that you are well suited to each other so as to look like a 'real' family, i.e. you have similar hair colours, the mum and dad are in proportion to each other, the siblings are a couple of years apart in age etc. You can expect to get all sorts of photographic work.

Freelance modelling – This is where you as a model will be responsible for

> **JEANNE'S TOP TIPS**
>
> STAY IN CONTACT WITH YOUR AGENCIES. A QUICK PHONE CALL OR EMAIL, EVEN JUST TO BOOK OUT OR ASK IF THERE ARE ANY CASTINGS. KEEP YOUR NAME IN THE BOOKER'S MIND. EVEN BETTER, POP IN FOR A CHAT OR COFFEE SO THEY GET TO KNOW YOU. THERE ARE PROBABLY SEVERAL MODELS THAT HAVE A DESCRIPTION LIKE YOU. YOU NEED TO BE REMEMBERED.

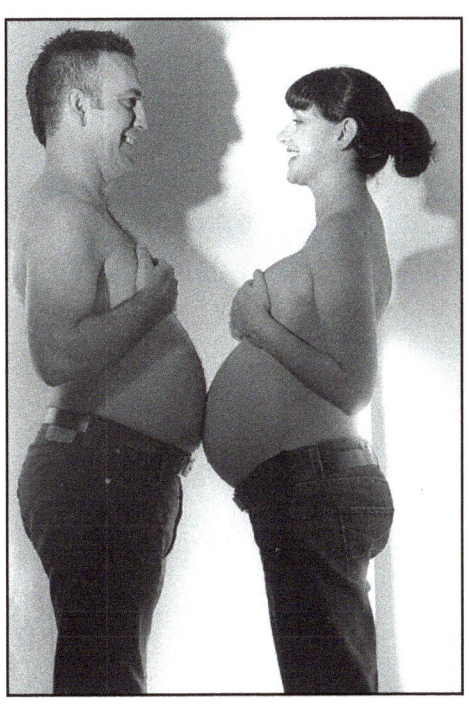

Tiffany doing pregnant modelling at 7 months.

Do You Wannabe a Model?

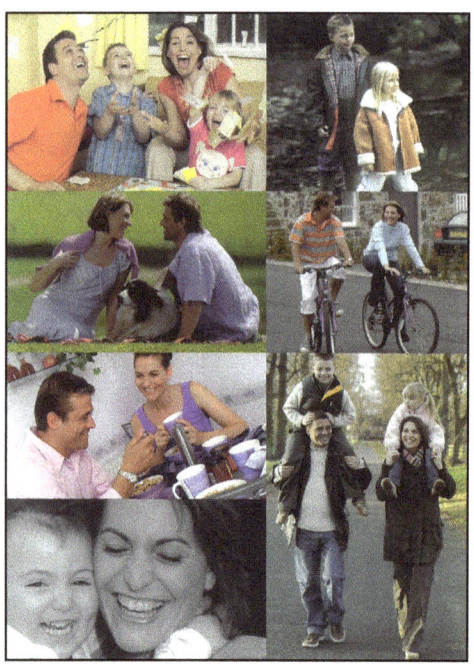

Sample of family pictures on a composite card (see page 57).

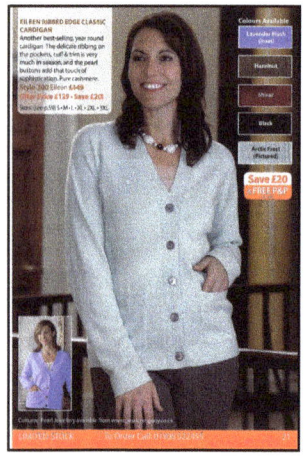

Mature/classic modelling.

finding all your own modelling jobs. Be very careful if you want to take this route as a lot of agencies will be wary of taking you on; they may feel threatened that you will take their client database from them.

Mature and classic modelling – Once upon a time people often thought as soon as you were 24ish your modelling career was over. Nowadays this isn't true – many older people are needed for all types of modelling jobs.

Photographically there are numerous catalogues that cater for the over 40s and this includes male catalogues too. These are full of clothing that looks good on an older person, yet isn't old fashioned or frumpy. Beauty products often need older models. Think Dove, which has just done a huge campaign in not only magazines but on TV as well, trying to show ALL generations.

Most advertising agents and marketing gurus know that the best way to attract their target audience is to reflect them. Senior models can be used by insurance companies to holiday companies specialising in breaks for the older generation.

There isn't just photographic work available for the mature model, TV and commercials are always looking for more classic models. This market has never been greater than it is today, advertising quality garments that suit a more mature figure and lifestyle.

If you are thinking of trying to break into classic modelling most agencies are not only looking for natural attractive models but also fit and healthy people who will have a better chance of getting work and fullfilling assignments. As we all know, ageing also comes with its own set of problems and ailments.

Types of Modelling

Other 'qualifications' you will need are to be confident in front of the camera and to not have any inhibitions. Good skin is an added bonus too – although not necessarily free from wrinkles or liver spots. This is a natural progression of ageing and companies may want to show this and, if not, liver spots can be easily covered with camouflage make-up and wrinkles can be easily *Photoshopped* out of a picture nowadays.

When applying to an agency (see page 24) send in a natural classic beauty shot and a simple full length photo. Don't try to be too young or follow any funky trends. They will want to see you.

Jeanne and the Liz Hurley look.

Lookalike modelling – If you look like a celebrity you could earn extra money by working as a lookalike. There are specific agencies that can get you lookalike work but expect these agencies, like model agencies, to take a commission. If they are reputable they may not be charging a joining fee but some agencies nowadays do charge an administration fee. You could look like anyone well-known, from the Queen to Elvis Presley.

Obviously people, like clothes, are fashionable, but if your timing is right you could do really well. Fees vary depending on the popularity of the chosen act. Also, if you are the only lookalike for a specific celebrity in your area, or even the country, then you can command your own fee and travel expenses could also be covered. You will be in a really good position to dictate what fees you want.

Another option, if you are a lookalike singer from a band you could try and find other lookalikes to be employed together – even better if you can actually play an instrument or sing, as you could perform together. Some lookalikes actually make a living touring the country doing tribute acts. If you are acting as a celebrity, in most cases, it will be up to you to provide all the costumes and accessories to 'copy' your chosen star, but this could pay off if you get lots of bookings. If you are a lookalike for someone who, for example, was in politics, you may have to study them from DVDs, film footage or news clips so you can copy their mannerisms and their little quirks. If you got booked on a job for a corporate event or video shoot you won't be booked for being you – they will not only want you to *look* like your celebrity but you will also need to *act* like them too.

If you sound like a celebrity you could get voice-over work. This could include radio ads, mobile ringtones or even SatNav voices.

There is always the option that you could represent yourself, but unless you have a lot of contacts or have been in the industry for a while, it's best to be represented by an agency. Below are a few agencies, but before joining them, find out first how many other people they have on their books working as the same act as you. If they already have several then it's best to try another agent.

www.fakefaces.co.uk

www.splitting-images.com

www.toplookalikes.co.uk.

HOW TO JOIN AN AGENCY

When applying to an agency you will need to write a covering letter plus a CV and either send it by post or by email. The letter should be concise – no more than one page long. An agency will have a lot of post or emails to read and won't want to read essays from wannabe models. Write a formal letter as this will look professional.

1. Your address, telephone number, email address and date should be in the top right-hand corner.

2. Write the agency address starting a line below, underneath on the left.

3. Find out the name of the person you should be addressing the letter to, which can usually be found on their website.

4. In the first paragraph state clearly what you want from their agency and the reason why you are writing/emailing – you want to be represented by them in their area. Explain whether you are an experienced model or just starting out. State the type of modelling you have done in the past and what you are looking for. Mention a few well-known clients whom you have worked for in the past, if you have this experience. Don't forget you are trying to sell yourself to them so make it interesting. If time-keeping is a good asset you have, tell them you are punctual.

5. In the second paragraph tell the agency a little bit about yourself e.g. if you are still in full-time education, or whether you have children. This will give the agency an idea about how often you want work or can work.

6. In the third paragraph state personal information, such as height, bust, waist and hip measurements. It's also an added bonus if you are a driver with a car.

7. Close the letter with 'yours sincerely' and by adding 'I would welcome the opportunity to meet you in person' so that the agency knows you are willing and eager to come in to meet them.

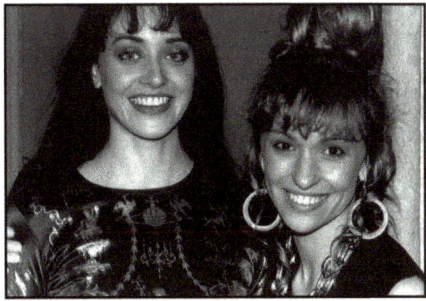
The night Tiffany won Miss British Isles '92, with Michaela Strachan, who was the compere and so lovely.

REMEMBER

● Avoid wording like "I have beautiful eyes," "my hair is stunning," "my mum keeps telling me I should be a model". These are all opinions and the agency will make-up its own mind!

● Everyone likes praise, so mention if someone has recommended the agency to you, or that you have heard that they are the best agency in the area, so you would like to be represented by them.

● Always get someone good at English to proof-read your letter to check for spelling and grammatical mistakes.

What is a CV ?

A curriculum vitae or CV is an account of someone's personal details, experiences and qualifications. A CV is sometimes the first item an employer may encounter about a person when considering an applicant for a job. The CV will be reviewed and it will be decided whether to take things further with an applicant, such as an interview. In the UK a CV is normally fairly short, covering two A4 pages, so it only really contains a summary of someone's experiences. A CV should be updated and made specific to certain jobs. Many CVs contain key words that an employer may pick up. All the content of a CV will be displayed in a flattering way – highlighting all the good points but brushing over information that isn't so great e.g. unflattering grades or exam results. Be honest on your CV but remember you should sell your positive points. You choose what is going to be put on the CV, so be selective!

YOUR MODELLING CAREER

The following section is full of information about all the different types of jobs you may do during your modelling career, beginning with Photography Work.

PHOTOGRAPHY WORK

Photography work is when a model is chosen to do a shoot for a company. It could be, for example, a fashion catalogue or a brochure for a dentist or sofa company. Pretty much anything!

> **TIFFANY'S TOP TIPS**
>
> BELIEVE IN YOURSELF. IF YOU DON'T, HOW CAN YOU EXPECT OTHERS TO BELIEVE IN YOU?

To do photography work, a model should be well proportioned depending on the trend or the market. A magazine could require a slim slender silhouette or a more curvaceous look. Male models should be athletic looking but not have the exaggerated look of a body builder. Proportion is always the key.

There are two types of photographic modelling. The first is editorial which involves jobs which appear in magazines and this includes covers. These do not pay so well but you do get good coverage and also get some excellent tear sheets for your portfolio. The second type of photographic modelling is commercial photography. Commercial photography can be shots that appear as posters in stores, billboards, newspapers etc and fashion advertising which are shots that advertise a particular product.

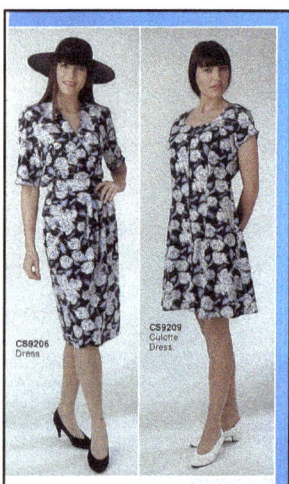
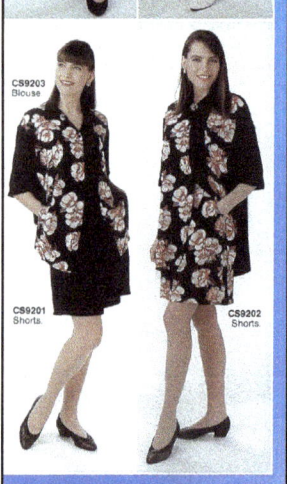

Left: One of Jeanne's first modelling photographic jobs. Below: Tiffany's first ever modelling photographic job at 18, working for her first agency Number One.

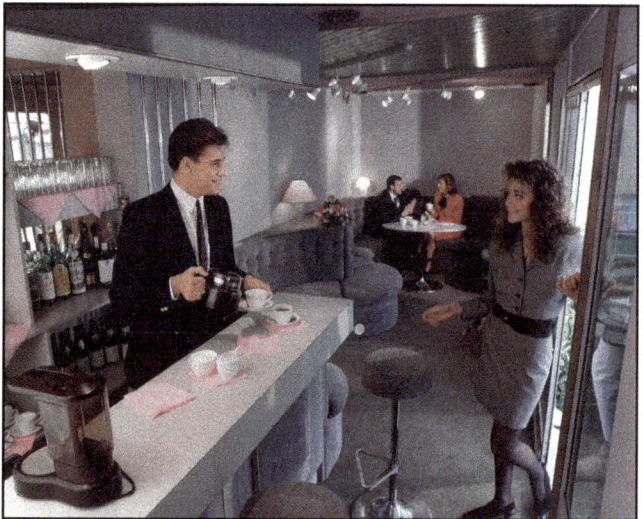

Photography Work

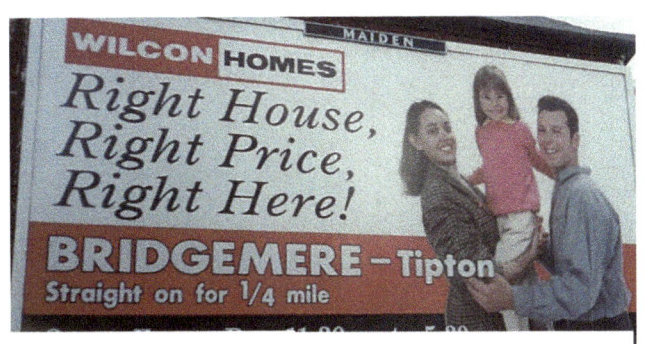
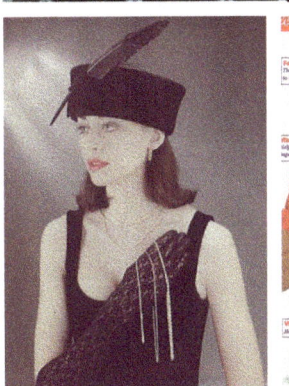
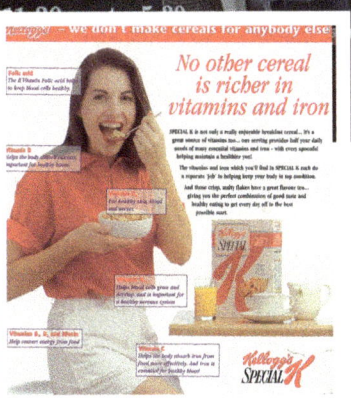
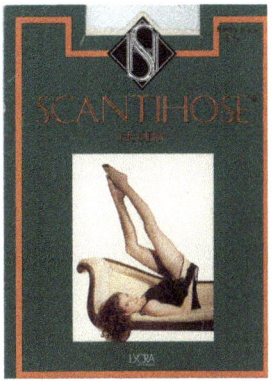

Left: Tiffany on a billboard. Bottom left to right: jewellery job for Tiffany, one of Jeanne's favourite jobs for Kellogs Special K and Jeanne's best paid job for Scantihose.

Photography work is often based on a 2 hr minimum (in most cases, but if it's a local agency you may be asked to do an hour), half a day (4 hrs) or a full day (8 hrs). The daily rates on average in Birmingham and Manchester are £60 per hour £200 for 4hrs and £300 for 8hrs. In London the rates are slightly more depending on the agency.

You may get a buy-out (see glossary page 108) fee which is extra on top of your day rate. You get this if the client wishes to use your shots for posters, internet, point of sale, national magazines or papers.

You may get a direct photographic job without having to cast, or you may have to go for a casting. Sometimes you may be required to do your own

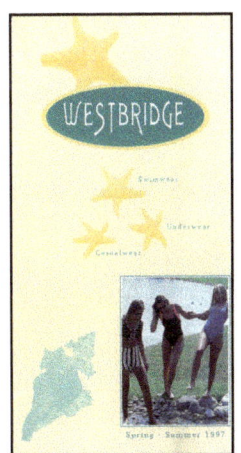
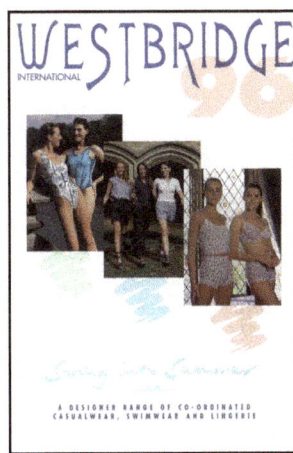

Tiffany and Jeanne both modelled for Westbridge but in different years. Left: Tiffany in the middle. Jeanne on the right.

hair and make-up. Occasionally a make-up artist will be booked on the job; you should find this out before you go to the job. When on a photographic job, expect the following to be at the studio: the models, photographer, photographer's assistant and client. Occasionally there will be an art director.

You may need to take your own clothes and shoes, or a specific wardrobe may have been sorted out for you. Always make sure your clothes are clean, not too fashionable, but classic. The client does not want their photos to date within a few months. Never wear strong coloured

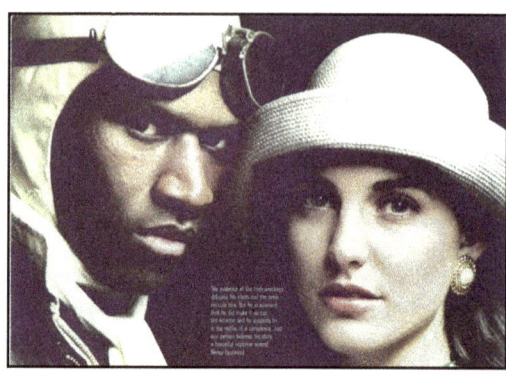

Jeanne's favourite work shot for a synopsis for a film.

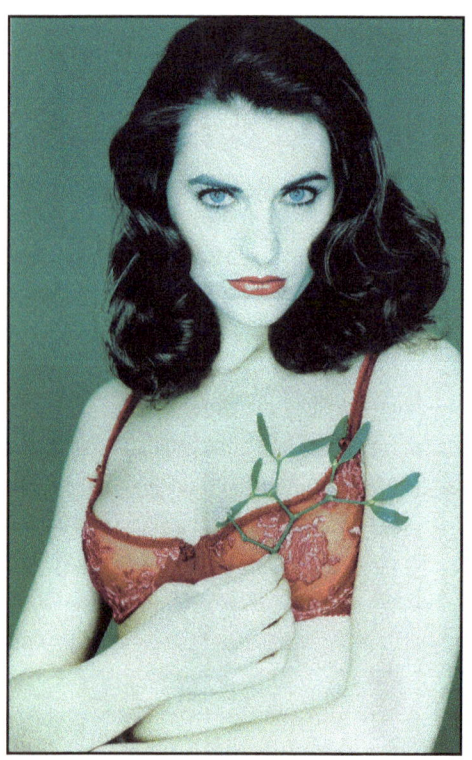

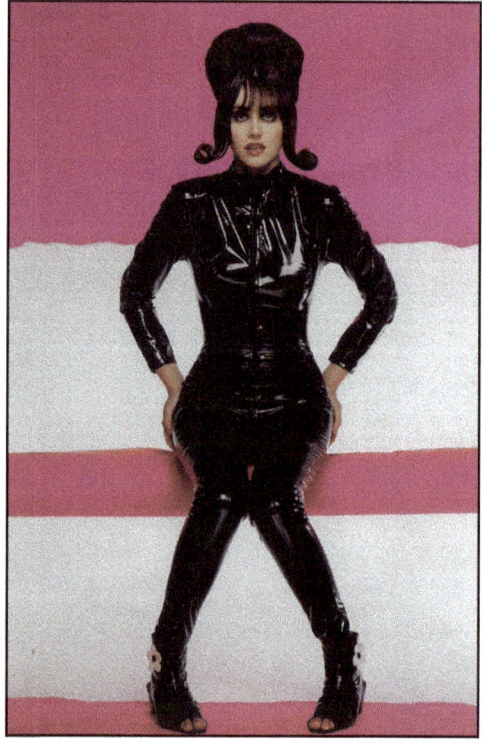

Tiffany's favourite shot of Jeanne – she looks like a 40s film star. Right: Jeanne's favourite pic of Tiffany, who worked with the amazing Umberto Giannini. Eat your heart out Betty Boo!

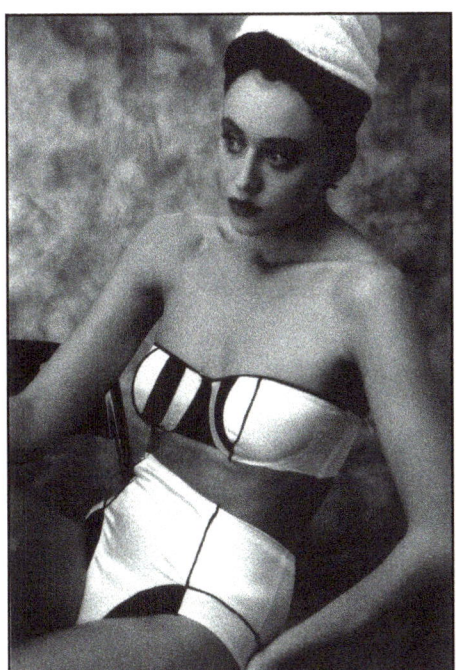 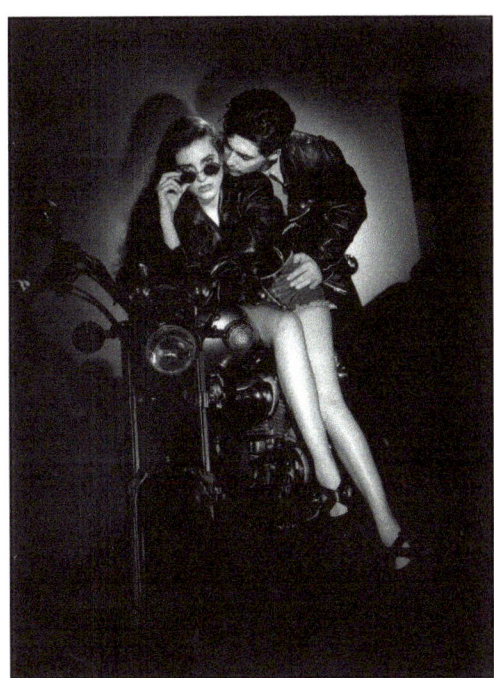

Left: Tiffany's favourite lingerie work shot. Right: Jeanne's favourite leg work shot for...Flicker Lady Shaver. I wonder why it's my favourite?

nail polish, a nude or clear is advisable. Never drastically change your hairstyle or colour after you have been chosen to do a photographic job. If you look very different from your promotional shots that the agency has sent to the client, the client would have every reason to send you home.

You can also get trips abroad for a catalogue shoot. Make sure your passport is always up to date. This is great as it is a block booking and can often be for four or more days in a beautiful country. Clients do tend to pay slightly less and you may only get a small fee for travel days, if at all. To save money the client tends to book the cheaper flights which are the flights during unsociable hours. Also be very careful when working in the sun as nobody will be happy if you get sunburnt. Always use a sunscreen and where possible, if waiting for a shot to be set up, wait in the shade. If you are lucky to get a trip abroad check when taking the booking what expenses you are entitled to. Who will be paying for your food? Are taxi fares included in expenses, and if you are parking at the airport car park who will be paying the bill? If the trip does not include your expenses you need to work out if it is financially viable to do.

Photographic modelling can be quite lonely work. Most of the time you are driving to the job on your own and you rarely work with other models.

DO YOU WANNABE A MODEL?

When taking a booking for a photographic job make sure you have written it down clearly. Always take a postcode where possible and a telephone number just in case. Most photography studios are in the middle of nowhere and are very hard to find. It is a good idea to call the photographer a few days before and get a few directions and whilst calling just double check on the clothing brief.

TOP TIP

TEN TIPS FOR POSING IN FRONT OF THE CAMERA

❶ Be confident.

❷ Vary your expressions – no client wants to look at lots of pictures with your facial expressions all the same. Try smiling showing all your teeth, smiling with your mouth closed. Also try keeping your face neutral but with your lips slightly parted. Get in front of the mirror and practise!

❸ Try tilting your face at different angles, not just always looking straight at the camera.

❹ Don't hold your breath – strange as it may sound a lot of people when doing their first photo shoot have a tendency to hold their breath, which can cause fainting! It also doesn't look attractive on the picture.

❺ Even if it's just a head shot you are working on still maintain good posture. Shoulders back, stomach held in. This will make all the difference to the shots.

❻ Don't hold your head too high.

❼ Don't hold your head too low – even the slimmest of people sometimes get a double chin!

❽ Be natural – if you feel uncomfortable this will be reflected in the photograph. No-one likes a stiff model.

❾ Try and control your eyes with the flash. This will take practice but if you are known as a model who blinks a lot the bookings will stop coming in.

❿ Make your eyes the windows to your soul – sometimes it's good to rest your eyes from harsh studio lights – close them for a second. Think of a thought and then open them as the photographer takes the shot.

REMEMBER

A photographer will always tell you if a shot is not working or if you don't look good. A sportsman can't just go out on a track, a lot of training and preparation is required. Modelling is the same. Shut your bedroom door and stand in front of a long length mirror. Practise positions that elongate your figure and practise your facial expressions to find out what looks good and what doesn't. Think carefully about what is your 'good side'. No face is symmetrical and if you have imperfections you can learn to hide these in photographs.

A LOOK BOOK

> **JEANNE'S TOP TIPS**
>
> ALWAYS MOISTURISE THE BACK OF YOUR HANDS. DO THIS WHEN MOISTURISING YOUR FACE. MAKE IT PART OF YOUR ROUTINE. HANDS ARE A DEAD GIVEAWAY OF YOUR AGE.

Originally this was a designers way of preparing for a fashion show or a photoshoot. This book was used to help make sure a model was wearing the right accessories, shoes, handbags with the correct outfit. As time has past these books have evolved for designers to show their collection today and are there to help people find out what is on trend.

HOW IT CAN HELP YOU

On a website you may find a blouse you love but aren't sure what to pair it up with to get the most out of the blouse. A fashion look book will show you the blouse as a day look making it more casual, and a more glamourous evening look. The blouse will be shown with possibly a trouser and on a different page with a skirt.

All these looks will have different accessories shown using a model. Some of these models have such a perfect fit for certain brands i.e. M&S, asos or new look that they will be constantly used by this brand or company or is called e.comm modelling.

The trends are constantly changing plus there are the seasons, Autumn/Winter and Spring/Summer so that it could become a regular contract for a model. Sometimes a model's face will be shown and other times the photographer may crop into the blouse etc.

FASHION SHOWS

A fashion show or catwalk show is where a model will walk down a catwalk to show off companies' latest products. These vary from lingerie, bridal, college shows or showing companies' new season collections. Normally the day will start with a fitting, which is where you try on all of your outfits and shoes to make sure they fit and suit you (and sort out which shoes go with which

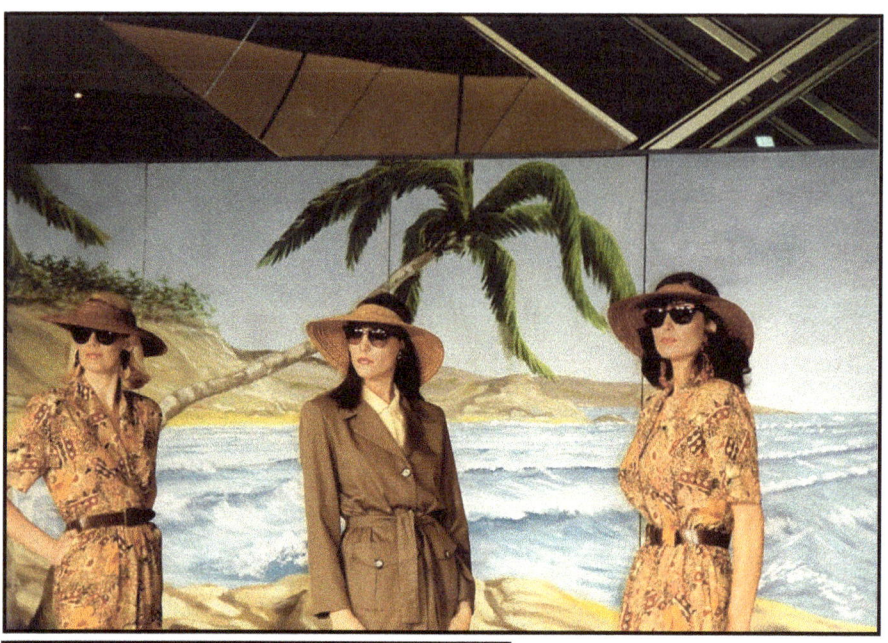

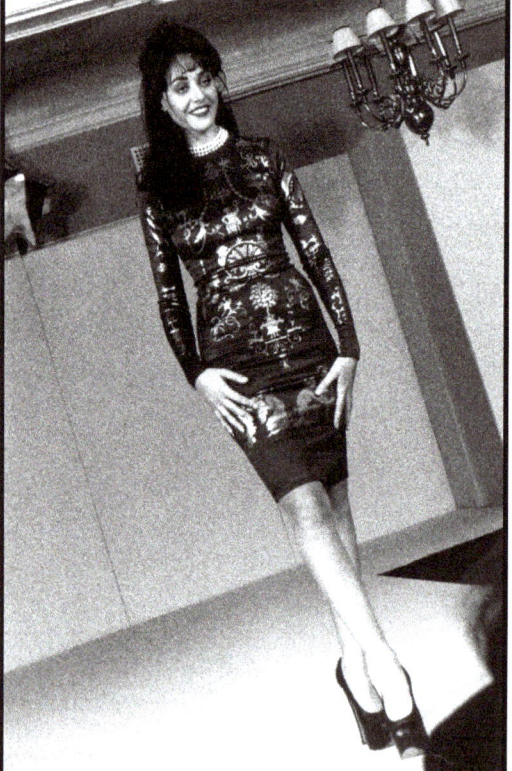

*Top: Jeanne at a fashion show at Merryhill, Dudley.
Left: Tiffany modelling Vivienne Westwood clothes.*

outfit). If something does not fit then the shop or client still has time to change the garment for a different size.

When you rehearse, the show may be a simple, straight catwalk show where there is no choreography. You will come on to the catwalk when you are dressed and walk to the front, model the garment and then straight off. In these cases you will usually go on to the stage on your own.

If the client has booked a choreographer, they will have worked out simple patterns or routines. If there are more than 3 or 4 scenes you will be required to write the routines down. In most cases a choreographer will expect you to count the music in beats of 8. When he or she says come on for one 8 it means get on the stage for a count of 8, then turn and wait at the back. They then might say to walk as a pair, go to the front and back for four 8s.

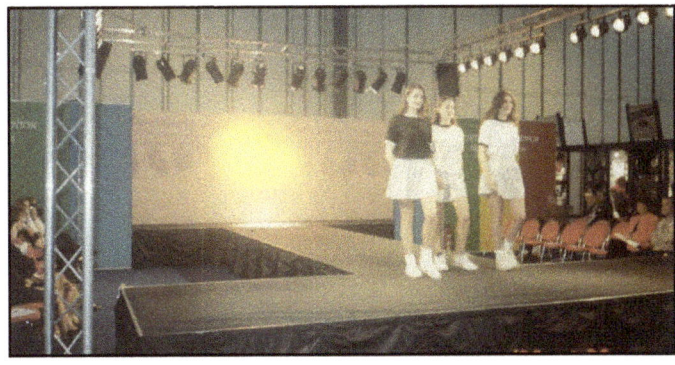

Above and below: Jeanne and Tiffany in a fashion show choreographed by Jeanne at the NEC.

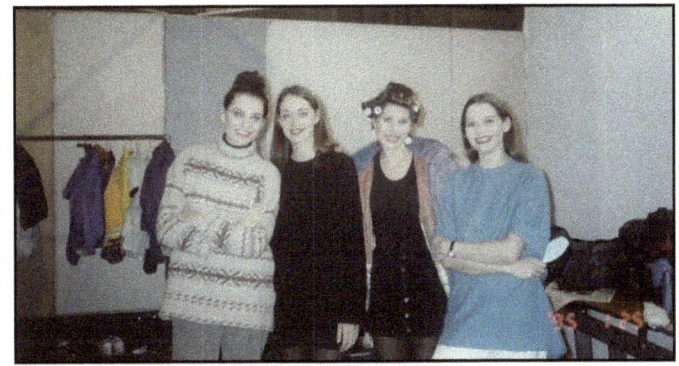

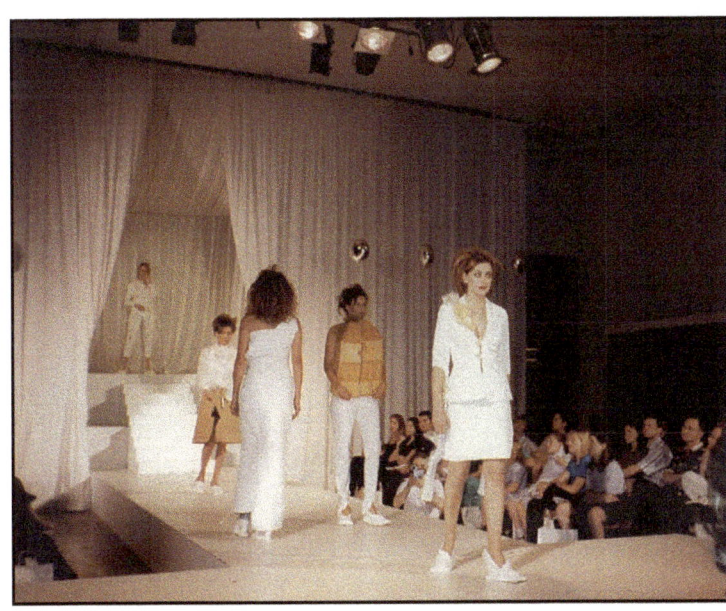

Tiffany modelling at the front in her collection she designed for her HND Fashion final year show.

Other simple catwalk steps to learn are:

Weave
Split
Waterfall
Cover the T / out to both sides
Peel out / peel in
Full turn
Half turn
Full turn, half turn together
Hold for 4 walk for 4

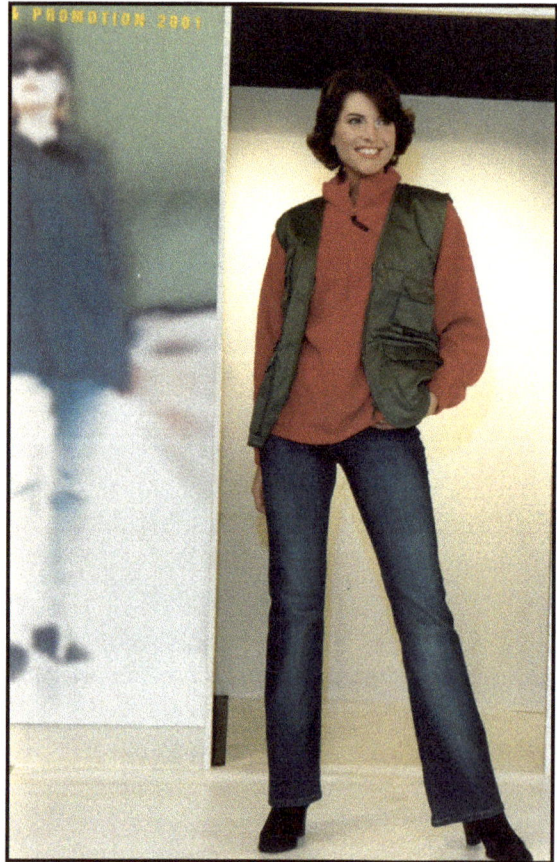

Jeanne modelling in a fashion show for leisurewear.

There are many shapes, sizes and heights of catwalk. Here are three examples: The T

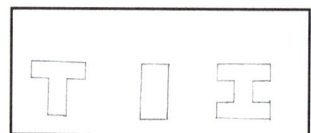

shape, The straight catwalk, The capital I.

There can be two entrances either side: you might have to use one entrance to come on and one to come off. There may only be one entrance. In this case you have to be careful not to walk into each other as one model comes on and one model goes off at the same time. If there are three entrances, which is rare, these are called stage left, stage right, and centre.

It is important to write yourself notes (to help you remember what scenes you are in) when you are in a fashion show, and you are perhaps in about four different scenes. When it comes to writing notes, make sure they are clear and concise. There is nothing more annoying than not understanding your own notes. There is no point in reading someone else's notes either; we all write our notes down differently and what works for one model will not work for another. Some models draw diagrams. We prefer to write it in shorthand. In between scenes you do not have much time to read your notes. You are too busy getting undressed and dressed again, sorting out your shoes and brushing your hair, so try and make it as easy as possible to scan through your notes. For example, if Jeanne was coming on the stage left entrance for one 8, down to the front for two 8s, out to the left side of the T and to the left. Then back to the middle for one 8, full turn for a count of 8, all the way to the back for one 8, where Jeanne meets up with model 2. Go to the front together for two 8s and then go to the back two 8s and Jeanne will go off the stage right entrance for one 8. To write all of this simply and quickly, Jeanne would write the following (as you do more shows you will learn a technique of writing notes that best suits you):

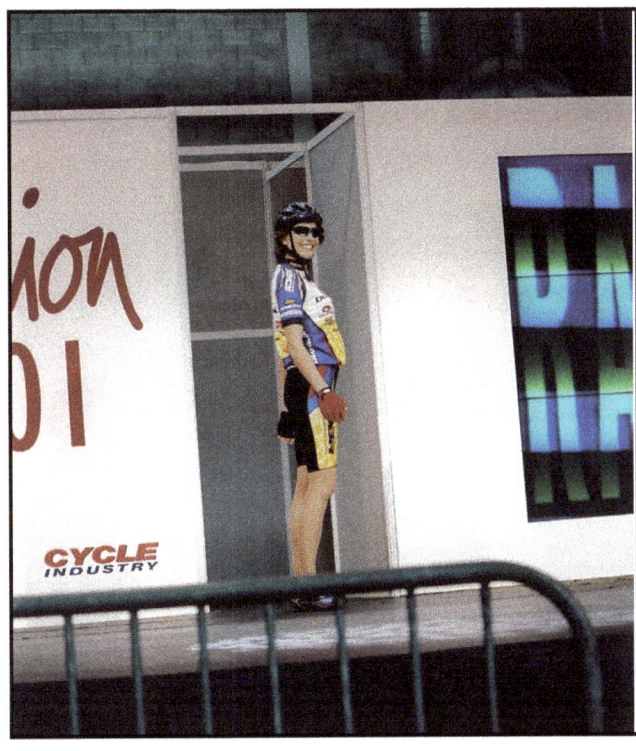

Jeanne in a fashion show at a cycling exhibition. You don't always get to wear what you want.

- SL ON 8   - 2 8s F
- Cover t   - 8 half way up catwalk
- Full turn 8 - 1 8 B
- Pick up   - as pair 2 8sF 2 8s B
- Off 8 SR

Do You Wannabe a Model?

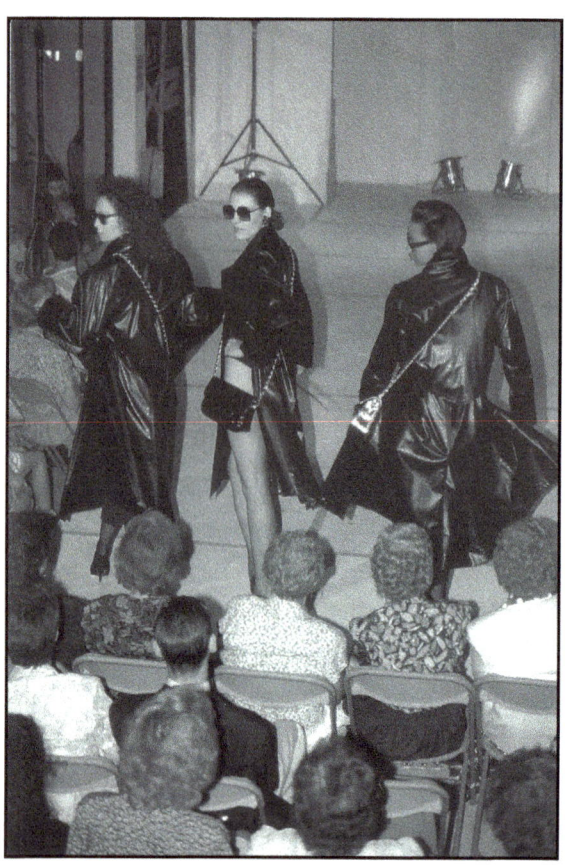
Jeanne in a fashion show.

All shows are different but on most occasions you will be working from approximately 9am to 9 or 10pm (this is if the show is in the evening). If it's a fashion show at an exhibition hall it will probably be a 9am-6pm day. You can get between £90 for a basic bridal show from 11am-4pm to £250 for a full day's rehearsal and an evening show.

Always take your model bag (see page 58) and make-up. If you are doing your own make-up, make it strong as fashion show lights can bleach out most of the make-up colours.

When taking down details for a fashion show job take down the address and always ask about parking as sometimes a boutique or company will have free car park spaces available. Always check that the address you have been given is also where the show is, as sometimes the fitting may be at a store, whereas the show is in the local town.

A RUNNING ORDER

A running order can be the order that the designers, shops or students put their show in. It may also be divided into themes, for example nightwear, lingerie, bridal or beachwear. It can be the order that the models go on stage, and there will be a running order for the music too.

A choreographer, or fashion show director, will normally arrange the running order and it will be discussed before the day of the show. This will allow everyone involved in the show to know what's coming next. Even the audience will have a running order in the form of a programme.

When you arrive at a fashion show everyone will receive a running order to work from, which will include the scene themes, models, music and any entertainment involved to ensure the smooth running of a fashion show.

PROMOTION AND EXHIBITION WORK

Promotion work is more in demand than photographic modelling, so it can be easier to get in to. You don't need to be a certain size or height for promotion work. Most of the time, if you have a great personality and are willing to work hard, the work will come flooding in.

Most promotional work is booked through a specific promotional agency. Occasionally a photographic agency will offer some promotional work too.

Most promotional agencies will need a couple of good pictures of you for their website. Whilst not essential, it does look more professional if you get a proper test done, and it will make you stand out from the other girls. If you really don't have the money, you could just send in a simple head and shoulder shot together with a full length shot.

If you build a reputation for being reliable and a hard worker, agencies and clients will remember you and will request you specifically for all of the best promotional jobs. This results in better pay and a steady flow of jobs. It is in your interest to show up on time and be ready to work for each event. Before responding to a job offer make sure you are free for all the dates. If you have a conflict, make it known up front, as this will save any last minute hassles. Agencies will book staff with the best availability first, as it is time-consuming and frustrating to try and work around varied hours and broken shifts.

For a promotional job you can expect to be paid between £80-£150 per day. A contract could be for a one-day booking or for six weeks, maybe on tour. Job types can vary from handing out leaflets in a local town centre, registering the delegates and handing out programmes at an insurance conference, to a drinks or cigarette promotion in bars or nightclubs.

Most promotional jobs pay within six weeks, but you do pay tax and national insurance on all jobs. If you end up paying too much over the year you will get a tax rebate at the end of the tax year.

On some jobs you may be given a whole uniform which will include shoes, whereas for other jobs you may be required to provide your own. You will at some point probably be provided with a promotional or corporate uniform that Tiffany's business Bareback Ltd (www.barebackfashion.com) has designed.

Do You Wannabe a Model?

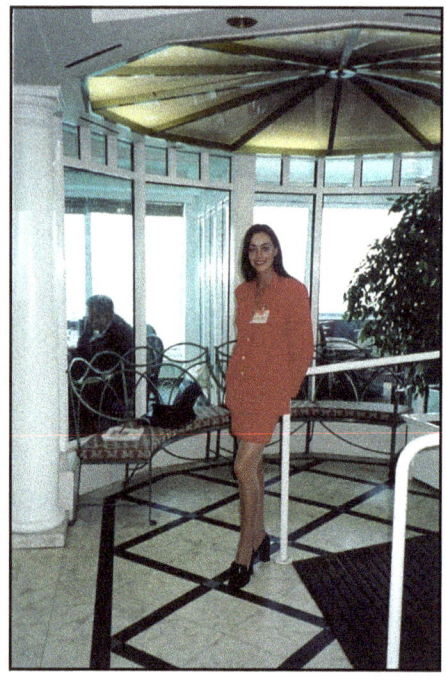

Tiffany doing a promotional job on the Orianna ship.

Some promotional jobs are great to get a contract for, for example The Motor Show. This is nearly two weeks of work. Most companies pay a reasonable day rate plus some expenses, and provide a uniform and accommodation.

Some promotional jobs are in the evening. This enables you to be free during the day and so you can spend the time going to castings or doing modelling jobs. The evening promotions tend to be slightly shorter hours but for the same money as a day promotion. It can be fun to do a bar or pub promotions as you get to enjoy the atmosphere whilst working with other people.

Promotional work is fantastic for the right person. You can make a great living from promo work and meet some fantastic people on the way. You get the opportunity to pick and choose which days and jobs you want to work on. You may even have the opportunity to travel if you manage to get a promotional tour around the country or abroad.

Even if promotional work isn't your ideal career, it is always a good place to start. This kind of work will help get your foot in the door

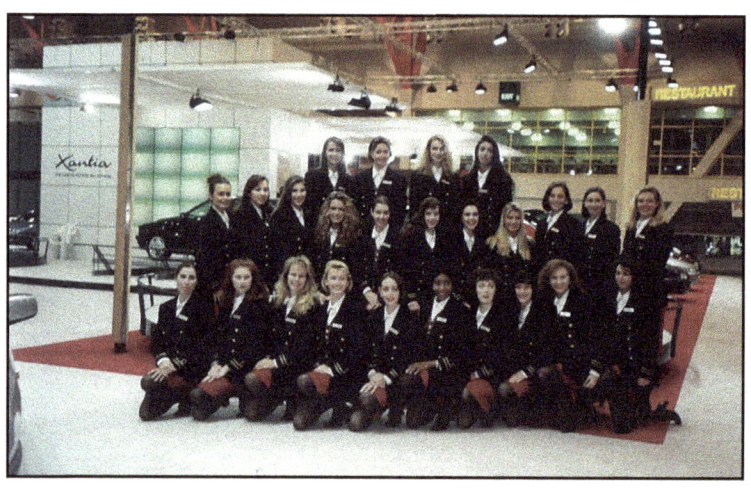

Citroen promotional girls at the Motor Show. Tiffany middle front row.

with modelling agencies. Also it's a way of getting some regular work to help pay your bills and will give you some money to test with some photographers. You'll also get some promotional products behind you, e.g. a composite card. It is a good place to meet other models, which is one of the best opportunities to find out which agencies are getting work and get and exchange some numbers. Some girls do direct jobs and get the work themselves and are asked to recommend other girls. If they have seen you at work and know that you are hard working they may suggest you.

> **TIFFANY'S TOP TIPS**
> IT'S OK TO MAKE MISTAKES: YOU ARE HUMAN. BUT TRY TO LEARN FROM THEM.

If you are very busy with promotion work and working for lots of different agencies it is a good idea to keep a clear, concise list of jobs you have completed and the dates and the amounts you are owed. You can easily get confused as to who owes you what, what you have been paid for and what is still outstanding.

EXHIBITION AND STAND MODELLING

A trade show is normally at an exhibition hall or centre, for example the National Exhibition Centre (NEC). They have these in all major cities and towns, for example in Cardiff, Birmingham, London, Manchester and Harrogate.

Normally trade show hours are from 9.00am-6.30pm and can show a whole range of fashion, from clothing, underwear and bridal wear, right through to hats and jewellery.

Some exhibitors will require a model and sometimes if the client is putting on a fashion show on their stand, more than one model will be booked. Most of the time a model will be booked and they will be required to try on outfits picked out by buyers of stores. The buyers will go through the range, marking out garments they would like to see on by putting a coloured disc on the hangers. The model will try them

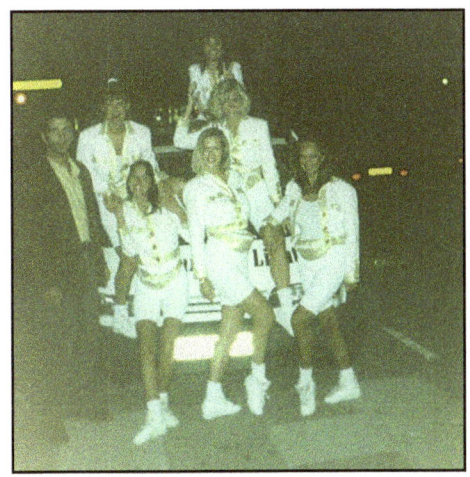

Tiffany front left during a six-week Marlboro Lights cigarette tour.

all on and the buyer will have a separate rail for all the garments they like, so they can look at the range together, after which they will write out an order.

This can be a hard job as it's a lot of changing, but it is regular work and there are lots of fashion exhibitions which include bridal, fashion, swimwear and lingerie, which can be held all over the country. The average duration for an exhibition is three days.

In most cases clients book a size 12, as most sample clothes are 12s, but as we all know sizes differ from store to store and this is no different.

Rates are approximately £140 per day for an exhibition and £200 plus for underwear and swimwear. Some clients will pay all your expenses i.e. travel, hotel and food. If you do need a hotel or B&B and you have to book it, make sure you do it early enough as local accommodation gets booked up very quickly if it is close to an exhibition hall.

PART MODELLING

It really doesn't matter if you are small in height (under 5ft 7") or a dress size 20 you, can still model.

Nowadays most of the big stores like Next and M&S have both petite ranges and larger sizes. There is a lot of work for girls who are larger than a 14. Models who are larger than a 14 are called plus size models. There are specific agencies that only represent girls who are plus size.

Most fashion shows in larger stores and shopping centres want a range of models. They will book an 8, 10, 12, 14 and 16 and will want them to be a variety of ages. If you are older there is work out there for you, but it is limited.

Part modelling is concerned with modelling certain areas of your body; just your feet, legs, eyes, mouth, torso, hair etc. You could actually just model your feet or hands on a full-time basis and earn a fortune, or model your legs for tights companies.

If you have a particular attractive part of you then you can model it. When you join an agency show them and do a test with a photographer showing that part of you so an agency can keep it on their books.

There is only one problem with part modelling: it isn't as easy as you think. If you are doing a photograph using just your hands and are holding a piece of paper, you will be surprised how heavy that piece of paper becomes after a considerable amount of time! It is always good to practise and this is why we test with a photographer. If you want to model your hands but you can't

Part Modelling

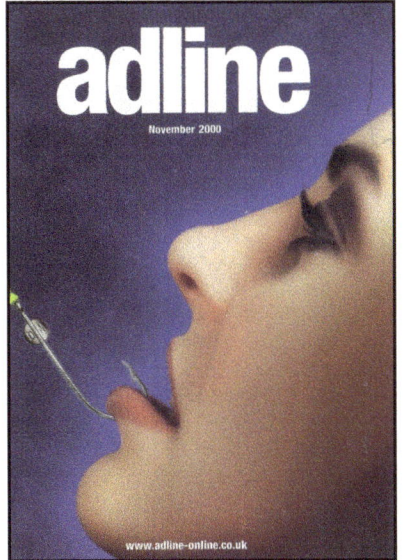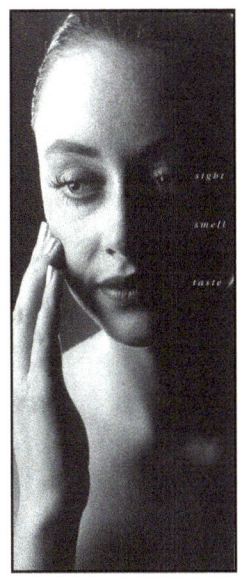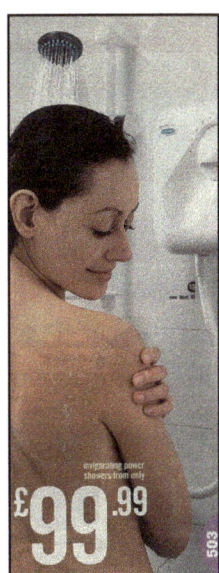

Left: Jeanne part modelling – looks painful. Right: Tiffany part modelling. The classic shower shot job. Got nude fee though! Below: Jeanne's lovely bottom and legs.

hold them up for an hour on your job you won't be booked. So be prepared.

When photographing one part of your body you may need to place it in very awkward positions to achieve a natural looking pose for the camera. You need to practise to get the positioning correct.

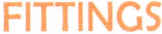 **TOP TIP**

FITTINGS

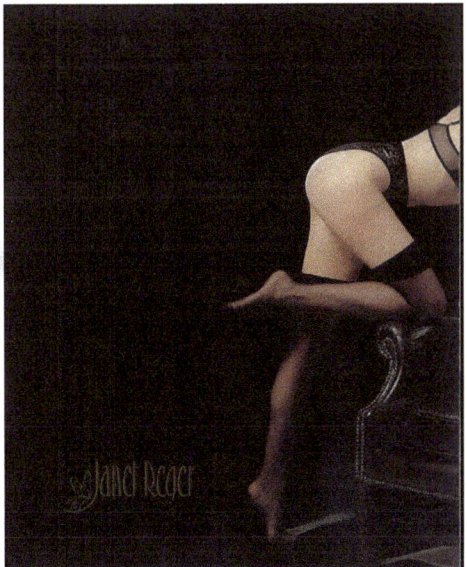

A fittings model, also known as a fit model, is used by a fashion designer or a manufacturer to check the fit of a garment, the visual appearance and the drape of it on a human being rather than a mannequin. A model will be

Do You Wannabe a Model?

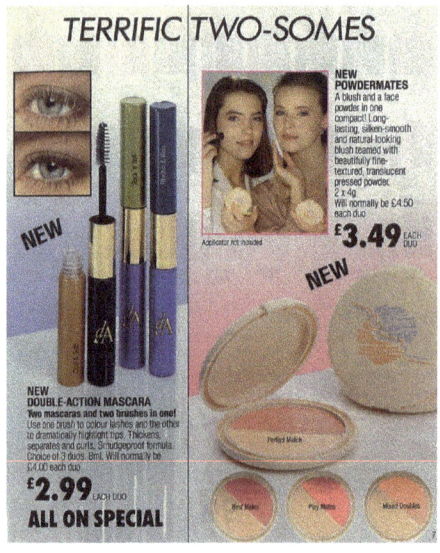
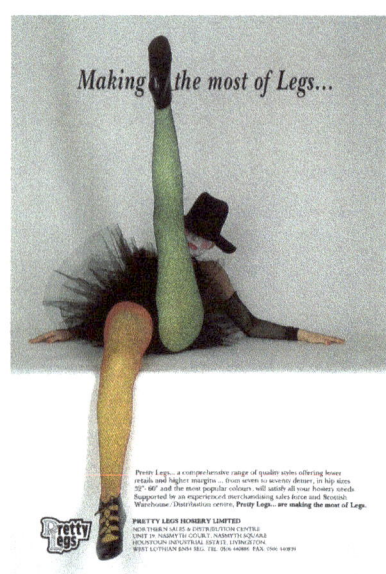
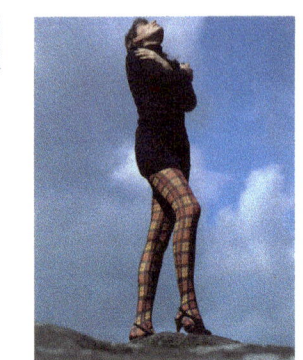
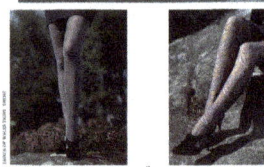
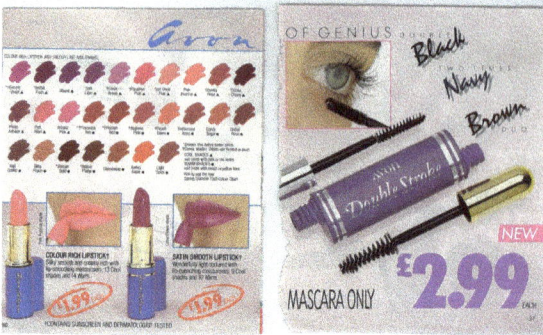

Jeanne part modelling and modelling for Avon. Jeanne modelling her legs. Jeanne modelling tights in a very awkward pose. Jeanne part modelling eyes and lips for Avon.

booked as a fittings model because his or her measurements are the exact measurements of the garments. These measurements generally consist of height, bust, waist, hips, arm and leg length, shoulder width and neck to waist. This is the same for both men and women and the grading of construction patterns is often tried out on a variety of fit models to make sure the size increases evenly across the range.

When working as a fit model you will only need the basic equipment i.e.

black shoes and natural bra and briefs. Whilst a designer is making a garment they could be designing it on you. A garment might only have one sleeve, a huge hole in the back, and may have pins all over it.

A fit model can become an important part of a design team commenting on a garment's material and general fit. How movement is affected when worn and the feel of the garment's material and general fit of something can be fed back to the designer.

A fittings model can get regular work and can make an excellent living, charging a day rate ranging anywhere from £100-£200 plus for underwear and swimwear. Obviously a fit model can't lose or gain weight. Some model agencies specialise in providing fit models and they are constantly looking for the perfect size 10, 12, 14 etc, a 38, 40, 42 chest for men, very tall, petite and plus sized models. NEXT, M&S and Asda are just some of the companies who use fit models regularly.

GLAMOUR MODELLING

Glamour photography is where a model is happy to pose topless or nude. Pick a job in this area of modelling with caution. Make sure you read all the fine print on a contract or check with your agency where exactly the pictures will be seen. Bear in mind that some of the bigger companies will not use you for other modelling if you have appeared in shots naked or topless, so make sure this is something you want to do, and don't be bullied into it. Make sure you will be happy and comfortable as it will be you standing in a studio naked in front of a photographer, make-up artist, assistant, art director and possibly several clients. Would you be comfortable?

Glamour modelling focuses on the model rather than a product being advertised or endorsed. Glamour modelling is photography where the subject, normally a female, is photographed in an alluring way. The subject may be fully clothed, semi nude or nude.

These pictures are normally intended for commercial use, which includes calendars, pin-ups and men's magazines. However, lingerie modelling can also be classed as glamour modelling.

Photographers will use a combination of cosmetic, lighting and airbrushing techniques to produce an appealing image.

One very well known glamour job is *The Sun* page 3. This does not pay great at around £90 for a couple of hours of shooting, but the coverage you get is priceless. The only real requirement for glamour modelling is to have a well

Do You Wannabe a Model? 44

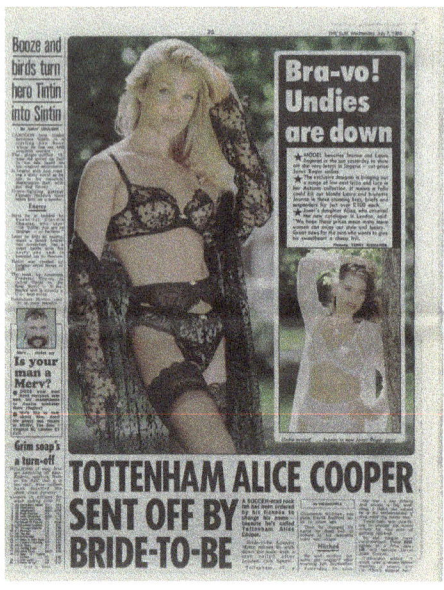

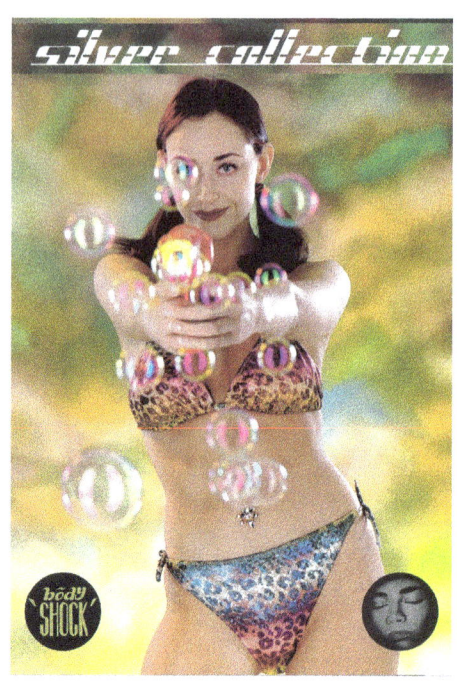

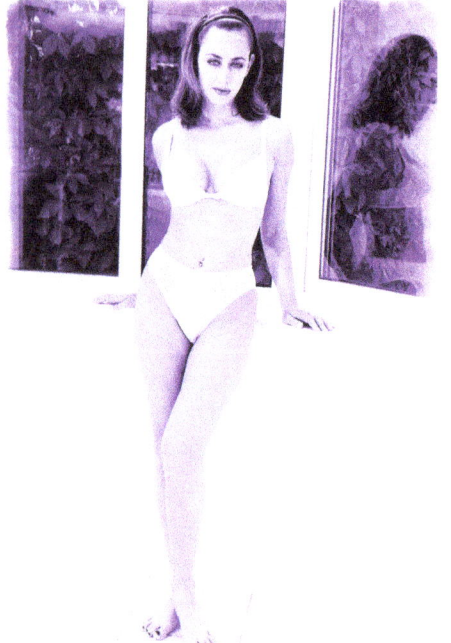

Jeanne on page 3 of The Sun. *One of Tiffany's favourite test shots – gosh I thought I had cellulite. Front cover wacky shot for jewellery company. Not going to show you inside the brochure...*

toned body. You don't have to have a huge bust or be a specific height. You need to be prepared to take criticism, which you have to learn not to take personally.

A great glamour agency which has been going for years is Samantha Bond and they are based in London. If you are interested in doing glamour modelling visit: www.samathabond.

net and click on their contact page. Here it will tell you what they require you to do to apply to join them.

WHAT IS A SHOWREEL?

A showreel is a motion picture (DVD or CD ROM) of an artist's portfolio. This can be some of the artist's TV work edited together. It is normally 2-4 minutes long. You can submit your showreel, together with a head shot, a CV and a covering letter. If you want to do TV work it is difficult for an agent to have an insight into your presenting skills from a head shot, so the showreel is essential if this is what you want to do. It can be difficult to get any TV work without having had any previous experience so anything which gives you experience is worth doing.

Some agencies may offer a TV workshop. This will help you with skills you need to have. At the end of the workshop you may even end up with a basic showreel as they will film you throughout the day. They may also be able to recommend companies that specialise in putting showreels together if you already have a few examples of your work. The cost of a showreel starts from about £400.

Check out www.theshowreel.com they have all different workshops at very competitive prices, including voiceover days and showreel days where you end up with a showreel. The starting price for this is just under £400. The showreel company is based in London.

VIDEO, PRESENTING TV AND COMMERCIALS

Being a successful presenter is a combination of personality, having a clear voice, confidence and being relaxed in front of the camera. However, it also requires other skills. For example a newsreader will be required to follow an autocue (a monitor near the camera which displays all the lines used when there are too many lines to learn off by heart). The benefit of this is that you don't need to learn your lines. A games presenter must have some knowledge of the game they are talking about, and a children's presenter must be able to relate to kids and keep them entertained!

When doing presenting work you may need to take orders from the director, floor manager, sound operator and cameraman. You need to be able to work under stress. You might also be required to work with an earpiece, listening to direction from someone whilst talking at the same time. This is not always easy! Most TV work is long hours: 10hrs plus, whether it's shooting a corporate video, a TV commercial or working on a show. You might also get modelling work showing the latest fashions on a shopping channel, where models are used regularly and can be paid anywhere from £200 for a day or £140 for a two hour show. Most shopping channel companies are based in London, like QVC, but there is also Ideal World shopping channel based in Peterborough. Most of these channels use models direct as the day rate isn't that great and booking through an agency will decrease the rate further.

Commercials are great to get – on most occasions the clients will cast. As well as getting a day rate you might get a buyout fee. You could also get a fee for certain areas where the commercial is shown e.g. the Midlands, Scotland or Ireland. Or you might be paid depending on how long the commercial is shown e.g. six weeks or three years. If the client decides to extend the time or areas a commercial is shown, your fee will increase. Some modelling agencies might get TV commercials or video work but if you want to get into TV seriously you might have to enlist a specific agent to represent you.

TV work is great to get but remember there is a lot of hanging around, it's long hours and most of the time you are on location and it can be cold. But the advantages are the money is usually good and it's great to see yourself in a finished commercial!

PHA in Manchester is a good agency which gets TV work like commercials and 'extras' for drama shows and it also has a modelling division www.pha-agency.co.uk

CASTINGS

In order to get to a level of success in either photographic or catwalk shows many clients hold castings. A casting or a requested casting is (just like in an interview) the one chance you have to impress a client and show him or her how you walk, or how you work, in front of the camera. Make sure you leave the right impression!

Here are a few simple tips to help you at a casting or a requested casting:

1. Make sure you are well groomed. *This reflects how you would turn up on the day. If you turn up scruffy, this might indicate what your clothes would be like if you were required to bring any.*

2. Be on time. *If you are late for the casting, would you be late for the job? Remember that you will not get a job just on looks and there may be a lot*

of other good looking people there. Remember: having a good personality and the right attitude is important too!

3. Wear simple clothes that flatter you. Wear clothes that best complement your shape. Do not be fooled into thinking that because you are tall and slim everything suits you. Ask a friend for some advice or an agency.

> **JEANNE'S TOP TIPS**
> USE KETSUGO, AN ESSENTIAL PRODUCT FOR PROBLEM SKIN. AVAILABLE IN A GEL OR SPRAY, SOLD IN MOST HIGH STREET CHEMISTS FOR ABOUT £12.

4. Keep make-up and hairstyles simple and basic. Do not overdo it by wearing loud patterns and colours, or going for a wild hairstyle, as this may not be what the client is looking for. It is best to be a blank canvas.

5. Be confident. Do not be intimidated by the other models there. There is a job to be got and someone will get it; why can't it be you?

6. Show Interest. Clients want to see you take an interest in their business without appearing overbearing. Ask the client a few questions e.g. how many models are you looking for? Where will the shoot be taking place?

7. Take your portfolio. Make sure it is presentable and not full of bits of paper but just your photos and a few composite cards.

GO-SEES

A modelling go-see is just like an interview and similar to castings. You can in any one day go and see several different clients all in the same area. This reminds clients about your model look and keeps yourself fresh in their minds. Just like castings you will show them your modelling portfolio, leave them a comp card and sometimes a CV. At a go-see (in London), you can expect to meet casting directors, art directors, photographers and fashion designers, amongst others.

Always make sure you arrive on time, are dressed appropriately. Sometimes you may get a call back (a second

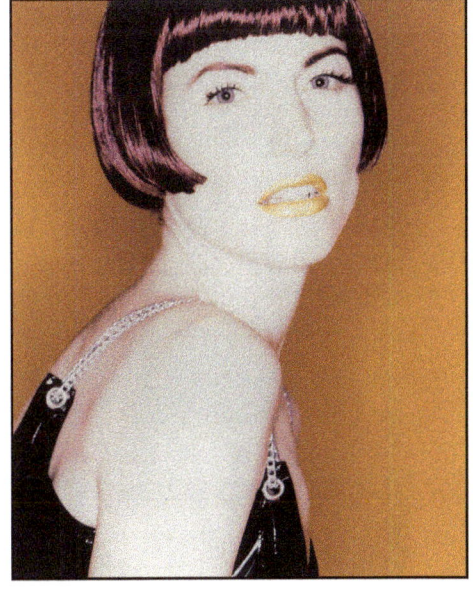

One of Jeanne's favourite test shots. Is that a wig?

> **TIFFANY'S TOP TIPS**
>
> THE WORLD IS YOUR OYSTER — SO GO OUT THERE AND GO GET IT!!!

go-see). This is when the casting director has requested to see you for a second time, along with a few other models who have been shortlisted, so they can then make their final decision.

ACCEPTING REJECTION

What is the most routine part of a model's life? The sad and honest truth is rejection. This is hard to accept and difficult to get used to but it happens a lot and is part of the job. You can not and will not get every job that you are put forward or cast for. From my experience many clients think models can't hear! We've heard things like "They aren't really model material", "She's far too thin", "She's far too fat", "Gosh, aren't her arms long!" and, personally, one that Jeanne had was "Gosh her hips are like a hippopotamus!". All this is said by people oblivious to you standing right in front of them!

You have to accept that you, and your look, will not appeal to everyone, and most of the reasons for your rejection will be for things you can't change, for example your height, the size of your feet, or the length of your legs. You need to learn to shrug your shoulders and brush yourself off and set off to the next job or casting. It's like a doctor being rejected for a job teaching primary school children. They are qualified for one job but haven't got what another employer needs. That is not to say they are not good at what they do. In modelling you ARE judged on what you look like and if you do not match the specification they have for the job, there is nothing you can do about it. Beauty is in the eye of the beholder, and what one person thinks is beautiful the next person won't, and clients aren't always looking for conventional beauty. Accept rejection graciously, but not personally. If you can't do this you won't last long, as this job will be too depressing. We all have something to offer and if you're not what the client is looking for, you will be what someone else wants.

The modelling industry is unpredictable – one minute curvy is in – tomorrow it's out. Accept who you are and don't give up at the first hurdle: try and try again. Castings are a perfect example of rejection. At the end someone has to get the job, but more than 40 people could be going for the same job as you. Even if your look doesn't fit for this specific job, you could always be remembered for another one in the future, so it is always worth giving it a go!

TESTING WITH A PHOTOGRAPHER

When testing with a photographer always make sure they are legitimate. Try and get recommendations from friends or agencies.

If you test with a photographer, most of the time you will need to pay him or her. Unless it's been arranged that you are doing a shot for the photographer, in which case he will do a shot for you in return and it's all free. You could go to your local college or university and see if any of the students will do a free test. You will need to be patient as they will take much longer than a professional and not every shot will be the best.

Rates for testing with a professional photographer are all different and can range from £35-£550. Some charge per look/outfit and others charge by the day. Most photographers nowadays work with a digital camera. This is great because you can get to look at your pictures immediately.

Once you have decided who to test with, ask to see his or her work, or check out their website. This will just confirm that you like the photographer's style. Make sure you know the exact rate they are charging and whether you get prints or a computer disc, or both. Find out how long it will take to get them. If they are giving you prints, find out what size they are. Most prints are 5" x 7", 10" x 8" or A4.

We would always advise paying for a make-up artist if you are paying for a photographer. This will cost between £35-£80. It will end up being money well spent. The photographer can always suggest someone that they have worked with before and you know that their styles will complement each other.

When you go for a test take a good range of clean clothes and accessories, and don't forget about shoes if you want to do a full length shot. Think about what your portfolio needs or is lacking. Take tear sheets out of magazines of shots that you like and would like to try and copy. The photographer probably won't be able to copy the picture exactly, but you will end up with one that is similar and you never know it may even be better!

Decide if you want to do studio or location shots. There are benefits to both: studio shots are clear and you are the main focus and location shots are great and interesting and can look like a commercial job, but there are negatives too. Studio shots can look similar, and with location shots you have to consider the weather.

If you want to get four looks from a photographer take at least six outfits. One of your outfits might not work, or the photographer might like your look so much he will be happy to do extra.

Do You Wannabe a Model?

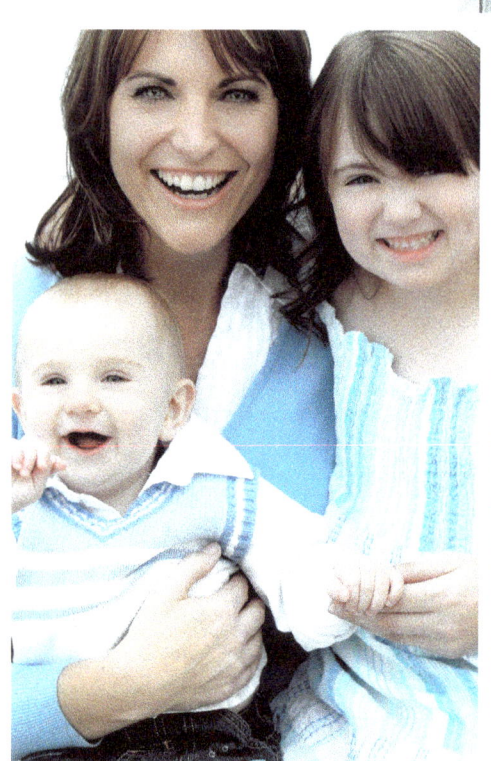
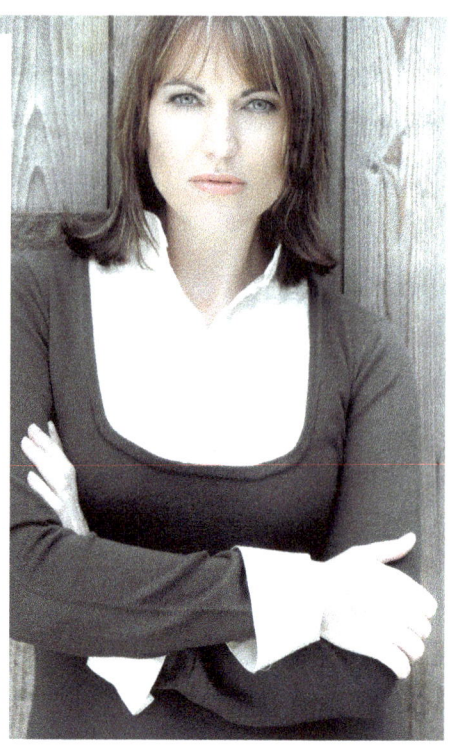
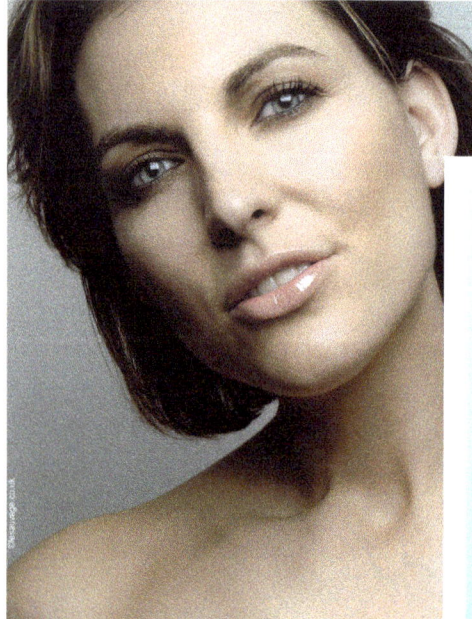
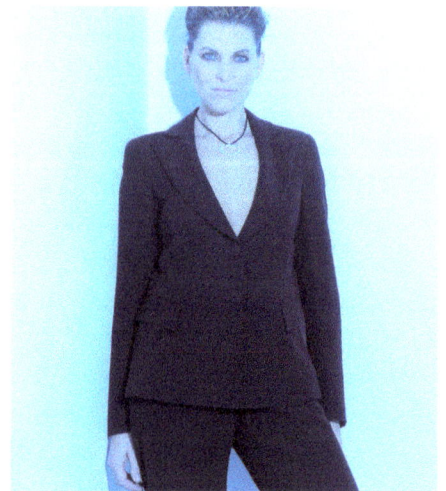

Some of Jeanne's favourite test shots. By Model Camp and Andy Lesauvage.

When you are an established model you will still need to test at least once a year. We all change in looks and it's good to keep the agency updated with shots.

Don't always test with the same photographer. They all have their own style. It's good to work with lots of different photographers so you get a variety of shots in your book which will show how versatile you are.

Be careful not to get sucked in by these makeover companies. They will often approach you on the street with a 'great offer'. They normally say the shoot is free but then charge extortionate amounts for prints. Some companies are legitimate. They provide a factory set-up which can be impersonal, and whilst you may be pleased with the photographs they can be totally inappropriate for a modelling portfolio. Makeovers are usually shot in soft focus, can be awkward poses and often date quickly.

CONTACT SHEETS

Contact sheets are rarely used now as most photographers and clients work digitally and this is often clearer. A contact sheet is a great tool though. All the shots from a test or a job can be seen at once and, through a process of elimination, can be used to work out which is the best shot. If all the shots

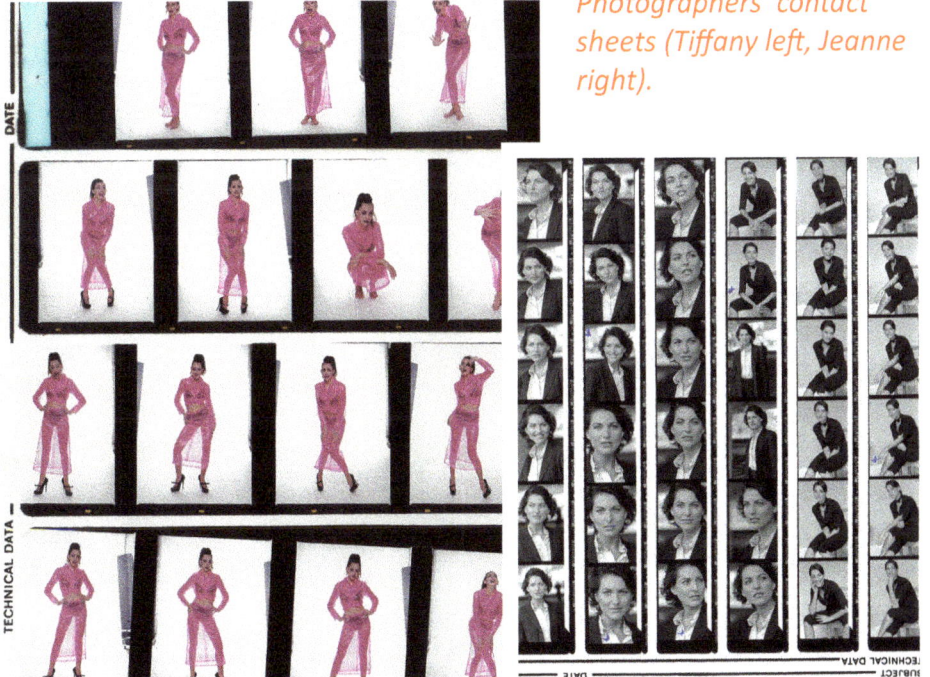

Photographers' contact sheets (Tiffany left, Jeanne right).

DO YOU WANNABE A MODEL?

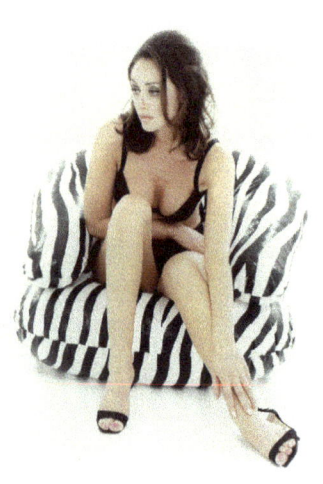

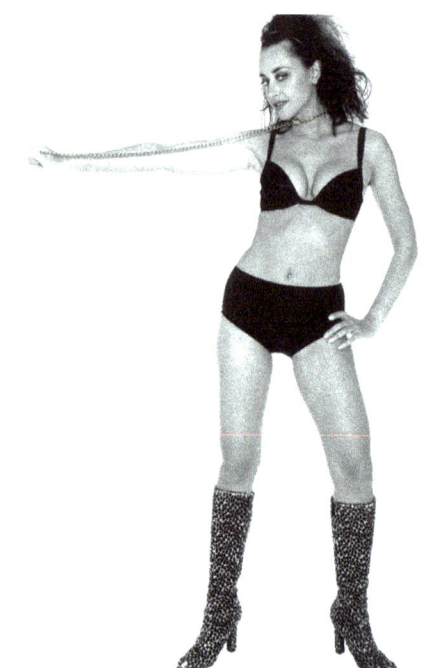

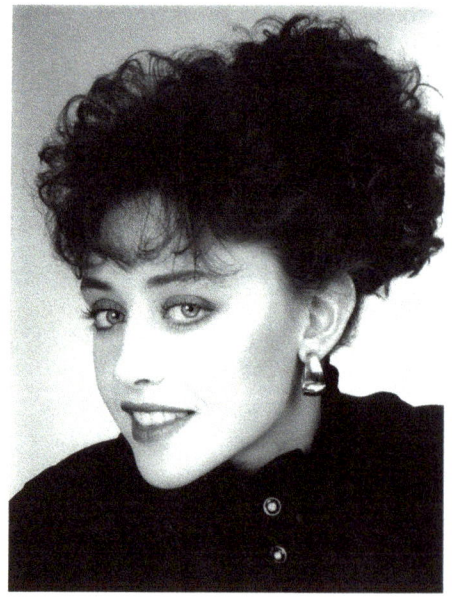

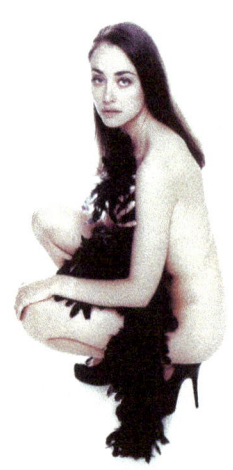

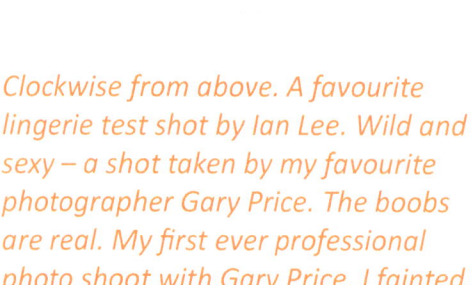

Clockwise from above. A favourite lingerie test shot by Ian Lee. Wild and sexy – a shot taken by my favourite photographer Gary Price. The boobs are real. My first ever professional photo shoot with Gary Price. I fainted. A student, Sarah, took this picture. It's another favourite of Tiffany's.

are great on a contact sheet you can use it in your portfolio, but remember what we said about pictures in your portfolio, don't overkill a shot! The picture size on a contact sheet is usually small so can be quite difficult to see. Sometimes a magnifying glass may be used to get a better idea of a shot.

PORTFOLIOS

After building up a good set of pictures not only will you have to show them to clients and agencies, but you will also need to keep them clean and protected. You do this with a portfolio case.

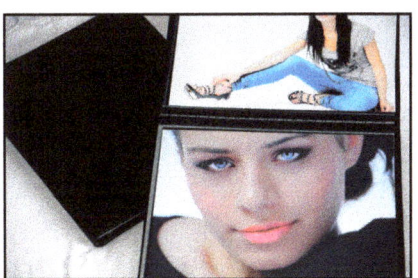

It is a good way of displaying and presenting your pictures in a professional way. There are many portfolios on the market but Wannabe Workshops sells an ideal one for the modelling industry. It is lightweight, black and sophisticated. It holds A4 prints perfectly and comes with 20 sleeves. It is also at a very competitive price which includes postage and packaging. Check out our website www.wannabeworkshops.com to order one.

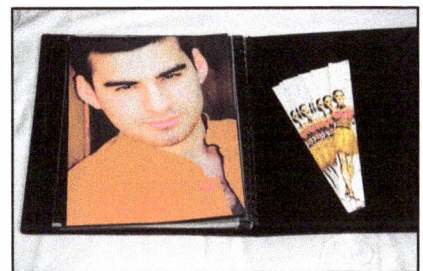

Here are the **don'ts** for a portfolio

1. **Don't** buy a portfolio that is heavy in weight – we have seen some metal ones which are totally unsuitable and very awkward. These are very difficult to carry round a city doing castings.

2. **Don't** have loads of pictures in the inside front cover pocket. A client doesn't want to open your portfolio case and have loads of pictures fall out. Keep it clean and simple and just have your composite card (a model's business card with pictures and measurements on – see page 57) in the front pocket.

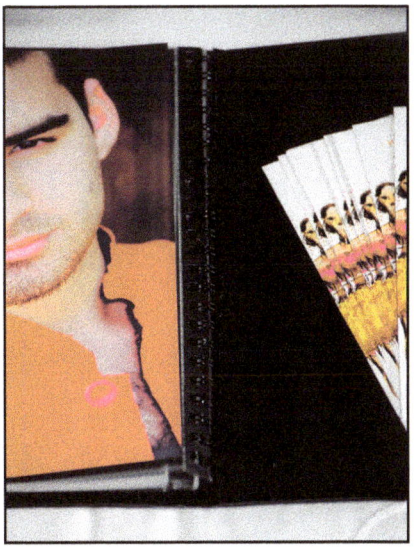

3. Don't have lots of prints from the same shoot. The maximum you need, or should have, is two shots from one shoot.

4. Don't be afraid of empty sleeves. Just because there are 20 sleeves in your portfolio doesn't mean you have to fill them all. Your portfolio should be a display of your BEST photos. It takes a while to build up a great book.

5. Don't have any agency logo on your book. If you join an agency and you buy one of their model books, what happens if you join another agency in a different city? Their logo is a way of advertising and not all agencies will like you promoting another agency at one of their castings. Model rates do vary from city to city and you could be reducing your rate if a client phones round to see which rate is the cheapest.

6. Don't get an A3-sized portfolio as your modelling pictures won't all fit neatly and it will look odd.

Your portfolio is a case or book full of sleeves or pages for you to display all your pictures. In some portfolios you can add or take away extra sleeves and some are like bound books. Tests that you have done with photographers and any work shots that you can get your hands on, should go into your portfolio. Keep a few composite-type cards at the front so when you go to castings the client can see them clearly and take one out for reference. Always keep your portfolio clean and tidy as it is a reflection of you.

Pictures that should be in your portfolio

1. Beauty shot. Just of your face, no accessories. A nice smile, but not a full laugh. This shot should clearly show YOU. It's simple and to the point.

2. Headshot. This does not have to be a close-up like the beauty shot. You could use accessories on this one such as a hat, scarf or maybe you could be laughing.

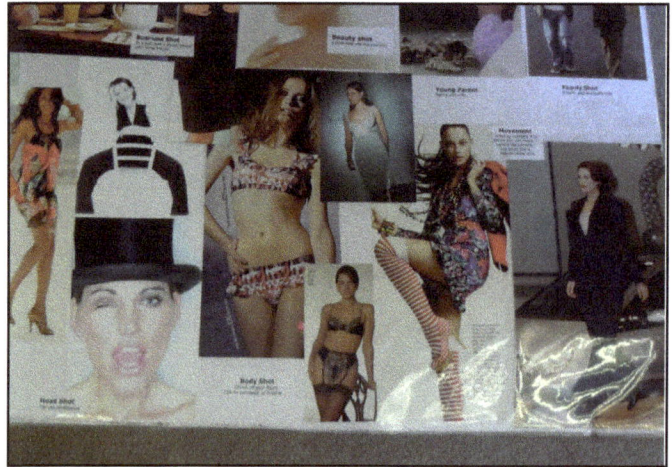

3. Business shot. This ideally needs to be taken with a suit on. Other ideas that have worked and been used several times before is standing in front of an office building, using a computer at a table or using a mobile phone. Wearing glasses is always a good idea to show versatility. You could use a second person in the shot to portray a business meeting.

4. Family. Even if you are only in your early 20s, try and do a picture with a baby or young child. Ideas for shots are: at a park, sitting at a table helping with homework, reading a story on a sofa or a child in bed with you by the side. If you are older try and find a male model that could work as a dad and do a walking shot as a whole family.

5. Full length. This could be fashionable and funky. Get clothes that are in fashion now. Get your whole body, legs and feet in.

6. Body shot. This is a shot that shows your figure off. It can be done with either underwear or swimwear. This is a great opportunity to show off great legs, a slim waist, and a good bust (not topless). If you have no interest in doing underwear or swimwear jobs, then a nice outfit that is tight and clearly shows your shape would also work.

7. Movement. It's great to see a fun, action shot: walking down the street, jumping in the air, running, or just turning round on the spot. This shows that you can move behind a camera.

These are the basic shots you need for a good portfolio. It will take some time to get them all. Try hard to get any work shots for your book, as this will show a client that you are in demand. I always think you can call a client once after doing a job to ask for a shot, then again a few weeks later. But I never call a third time. This can be pestering and at the end of the day you did the job and got paid for it. You are not entitled to a shot, but they are valuable.

It is vital to have a range of *different* looks in your portfolio to show your versatility. If you were on a casting for Boots' mother and baby range and all your photographs were fashionable, single shots, a client might find it difficult to imagine you in a mother role.

Even if you have 20 pages in your portfolio, you do not have to fill them all. Choose wisely and ask others in the industry for their opinion. In the

> **JEANNE'S TOP TIPS**
>
> ALWAYS TRY YOUR BEST ON EVERY JOB – EVEN IF YOU REALLY DON'T PERSONALLY LIKE WHAT YOU ARE DOING OR WHO YOU ARE WORKING WITH. IT IS BETTER TO BE IN THE POSITION TO BE THE ONE THAT TURNS A JOB DOWN, RATHER THAN NOT BEING REBOOKED. YOU NEVER KNOW WHAT POSITION YOU MAY BE IN, FINANCIALLY, IN THE FUTURE. YOU MAY REALLY NEED THE WORK.

end if you only have 10 fantastic pictures in your book, this is better than having 10 pictures that get lost in a book of 20 OK pictures.

MINI BOOK

A mini book is basically a smaller version of your current modelling portfolio. It will all be printed to an A5 size, including the size of the portfolio case and will be permanently kept at your model agencies office.

The mini book will have your name, height, body measurements and specialities on the front cover, so that they can be seen easily by the agency's clients. The reason for a mini book is that on occasions you might not be available to meet certain clients who have requested to see you, because you are at castings, go-sees or doing a modelling job.

A DISC

A disc is what a photographer may give you a few days after your test. This is great as you can see all of the shots on your computer at home before you buy any prints. Many of the photographers who work with a digital camera can re-touch some of the pictures and this will be included in the test fee. If you have a stray hair or a spot on the day of the shoot (and we all get them!) it can be erased on the computer. But be careful! If too much of your photograph has been digitally enhanced, the photograph may not be a true representation of you. Many clients will not be pleased if they are expecting a specific look to walk through the door and someone else looking totally different turns up!

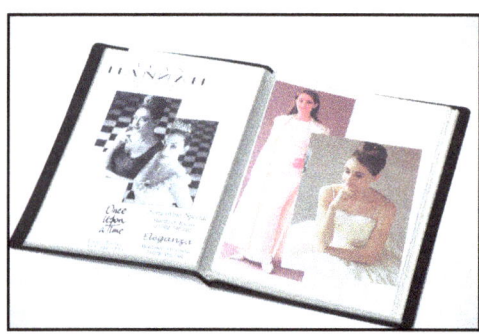

Sample of a mini book.

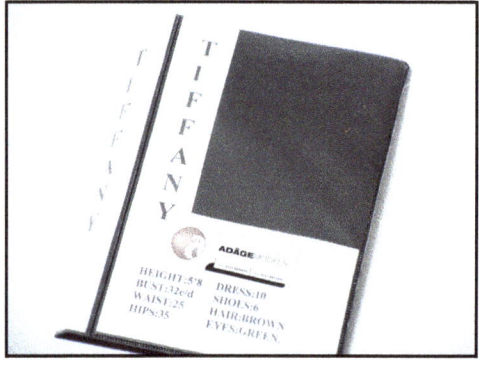

It is best to get your pictures as a jpeg format. Once you have a digital format you can print your own prints if you have a printer at home or you can do it through an online processor.

One real bonus of digital format is that you can attach your pictures to an email and send them out for jobs and to agencies. It is easy to do at the click of a button, but be careful not to send too many attachments, as they will take forever to download.

TIFFANY'S TOP TIPS

ALWAYS TAKE YOUR MAKE-UP OFF BEFORE YOU GO TO BED, AND WEAR A GOOD NIGHT MOISTURISER.

COMPOSITE CARD

A composite card, also know as a comp card, is a marketing tool for models. It showcases the best of a model's portfolio and is used as a business card. A comp card typically consists of two sides which have a cover with a full size portrait, and on the other side a selection of shots from the model's portfolio.

All the model's statistics will also be on it, including the height, bust, waist, hips, shoe size, inside leg length, hair and eye colour. For men this would also include a collar and jacket size. Any special skills that you have e.g. underwater swimming, ballroom dancing or horse riding should also be mentioned here.

The comp card is normally printed on a thick card approximately six inches in width by eight inches in length. It can be printed in either colour or black and white and can be a single or double card. Comp cards can vary in price depending on the quantity you have printed, the number of pictures you use, the type of card and the general print quality. All different layouts and styles are available.

Your model agency will always help you with your comp card, especially when you are starting your career. They should give you advice on what market you should appeal to and which looks and images best suit you.

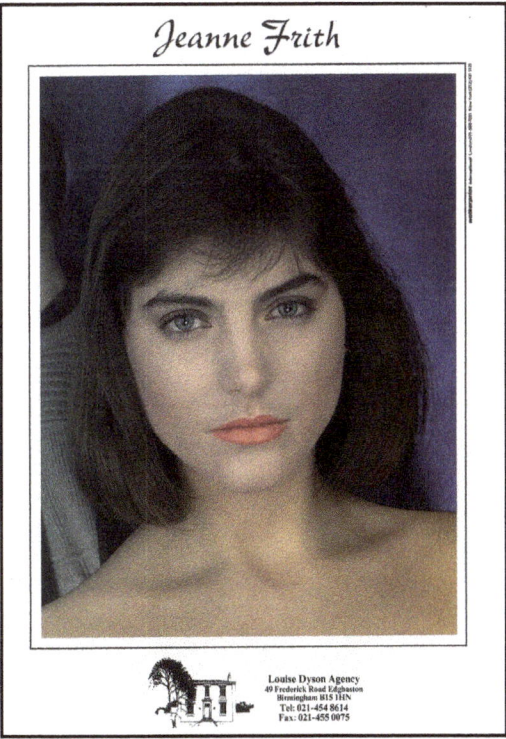

Jeanne's first model comp card.

Do You Wannabe a Model?

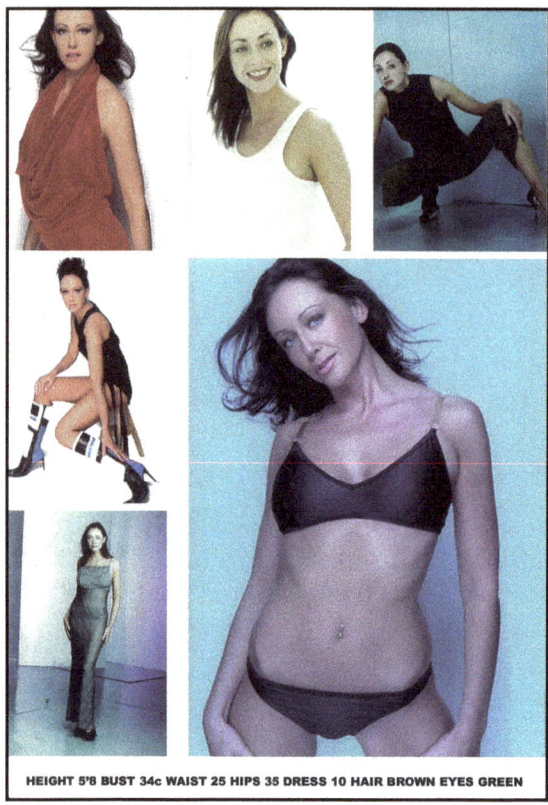

HEIGHT 5'8 BUST 34c WAIST 25 HIPS 35 DRESS 10 HAIR BROWN EYES GREEN

Tiffany's last ever comp card.

Useful website addresses for composite card printers:

www.imex-print.co.uk offers free proofs and free delivery.

www.centreprint.co.uk offers free proofs and free delivery.

www.doyourprint.co.uk has templates to create your own card using your pictures.

MODEL BAG

A model bag is a bag full of your own things for a job. It has a basic range of accessories that you might need on any photographic job or fashion show. Your bag MUST include the basics below. If you have anything that is currently on trend, take it, but ensure you have the basics.

Female:

1. Shoes – a classic style, for example a timeless stiletto (any shoe that is too trendy will date a photograph). Basic colours should include: black, navy, brown, white/cream, pewter, gold/silver and black or brown boots. Tip: Have shoes you only use for work and separate shoes for everyday use. This will ensure your work shoes never look worn and tatty.

2. Tights – a range of natural and black sheer tights. In winter have opaque tights.

3. A strapless, natural bra and briefs.

4. A petticoat, as some summer dresses can be sheer.

5. Hair accessories: straighteners, rollers, hair bands, grips and hairspray.

6. Simple accessories: e.g. diamond or pearl studs.

7. Lightweight dressing gown.

Male:

1. Basic black and brown shoes and trainers.
2. Black smart flat boot/work boot: e.g. Timberland.
3. Black socks and white socks.
4. Black underwear and white underwear.
5. Jockstrap if underwear or swimwear is being modelled.
6. Black cufflinks.
7. A black and a brown belt.
8. Make-up: translucent face powder, touché éclat undereye stick and spot cream.
9. Oil and body lotion if shooting a body shot.
10. Hand cream if modelling hands.
11. Various hair products – gels and waxes.
12. Lightweight dressing gown.

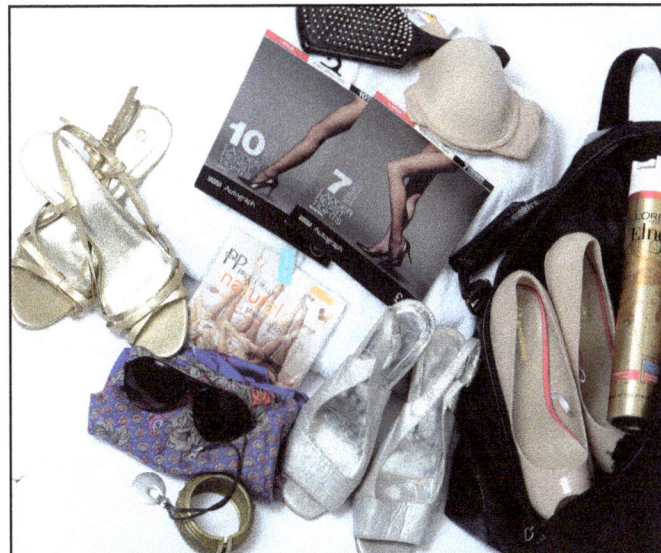

Inside a typical model bag.

When the agency gives you the details for a job they will give you a list of equipment to bring. Always try and take a bit more than they ask for. Take your portfolio on every photographic job if it's the first time you have worked with the photographer. It is always good to promote yourself and you never know, they may have another job the following week and you may fit the requirements for that job too.

DIRECT BOOKING

At any point you could be asked to do a job direct for a client. This means you will need to sort out all the arrangements yourself, the address of the job, right down to the fee with the client. Work on the principle that by

An example of a model release form.

doing direct work *you* will get slightly more money and the *client* will pay slightly less. Never agree a fee with a client and then go back and tell them you want more. This will only make you appear unprofessional and the client may have worked out the whole budget of the shoot on the rate you initially quoted. Always arrange terms of payment (when and how you will get paid) before the job i.e. payment on the day, or within 30 days of the invoice. Make sure you have included travel. Discuss with the client what the shots will be used for and include a buyout fee if there is a lot of promotional material i.e. point of sale, website, newspapers etc. An example of an invoice is on page 108 but you can get invoice books from any stationary shop like WHSmith.

A MODEL RELEASE FORM

You may be required to sign a model release form when you are working on a photographic job. Before signing it always check with your agency and make sure it has been agreed by them. Signing this document means that if the client decides to use your pictures for any other promotional material other than that agreed by your agency you will not be entitled to any more money. Most clients will know this and may try to get you to sign it, trying to make it look like it is no big deal. If in doubt always ASK your agent.

INVOICES

An invoice or bill is a document issued by you to an agency or client, indicating the agreed prices for modelling services that you have provided to the purchaser. An invoice indicates that the purchaser must pay the model, according to the agreed payment terms. The purchaser usually has a maximum amount of days to pay for these services. An invoice usually specifies quantity, price, discount and duration of modelling services. Generally speaking, each line of a rental invoice will state the actual hours, days, weeks, months, for which payment is required. An example of an invoice is on page 108 at the back of this book but you can get invoice books from any stationary shop like WH Smith.

DOS AND DON'TS OF MODELLING

A list of simple rules to follow:

Dos

1. Always be professional and on time for a job.

2. Make sure you have all the details written down for a job including how much you will come out with after commission has been taken off.

3. Join a reputable agency.

4. Always test with a recommended photographer.

5. If you are taking clothes to a job make sure they are clean and ironed. A photographer may have someone who can give a little press to a garment but they don't want to be there for ages ironing your weekly laundry.

6. If you get the time, pop into your agency to say "hi" regularly. This will always keep you in their minds. Some agencies have hundreds of people on their books and you need to stand out.

7. Inform a client or your agent in advance if you are unable to provide any clothes/accessories that they have requested.

Don'ts

1. **Never ever** pay to register with an agency. No joining fee should ever be charged if it is a good modelling agency. Nowadays an agency may charge you an administration fee.

2. Don't put yourself in a vulnerable situation. If you feel uncomfortable with something you are asked to do, or feel unsafe, leave and inform your agency. If you are under 16 and testing with a photographer it is always wise to take an adult with you.

3. Never pay huge amounts of money for photographers who claim they will give you a portfolio. Spend your money wisely.

4. Don't pay for a huge number of prints. You only need one or two prints of any particular look in your book.

5. Don't keep pestering a client for work shots. Call twice maximum. Remember, you have been paid for the job and are not entitled to any shots.

6. Never say you can do something if you can't e.g. ride a horse or roller skate. You will be found out!

7. Never 'steal' agencies' clients. You will, over time, build up a direct client list of your own, if you are a good model.

Note – All agencies will have a list of their own 'Dos and Don'ts' that they will expect you to follow when joining/representing them.

MODELLING SCAMS

Really it is difficult to find out if something is a scam without doing it first, which is time-consuming and costly and the reason why Tiffany and I set up Wannabe Workshops to start with. As time goes on you will learn by your mistakes. The basic things to remember are to steer clear of anybody who wants to take any money off you to join their agency, or charge you to go to auditions or castings. Any reputable agencies do not charge you anything to join them. Never answer an advert in a local paper; we have heard a lot about these from parents who come on our Wannabe Workshops and have been the victims of these scams. Tiffany and I have fallen for the paper scams over the years too. There are so many helpful websites on the internet and you can never do too much research. Before signing up for anything check by using Google and then check again. In the end you will know in yourself whether it sounds a legitimate deal. If they are promising you the earth nine times out of 10 it will be a scam.

Modelling is a profession where there are no text book answers. You don't have to have any qualifications and you can't go to university to study it, and although there are numerous versions of Wannabe Workshops holding model courses, no one can guarantee work as a model like an apprenticeship electrician course can.

Basically, models do not have a voice. There is no organisation that will make sure that models get the right amount of pay, that an agency can't hold on to a model's money for an unreasonable amount of time or that a model isn't pressurised into doing a topless or nude shot when they are at a job, worried that if they

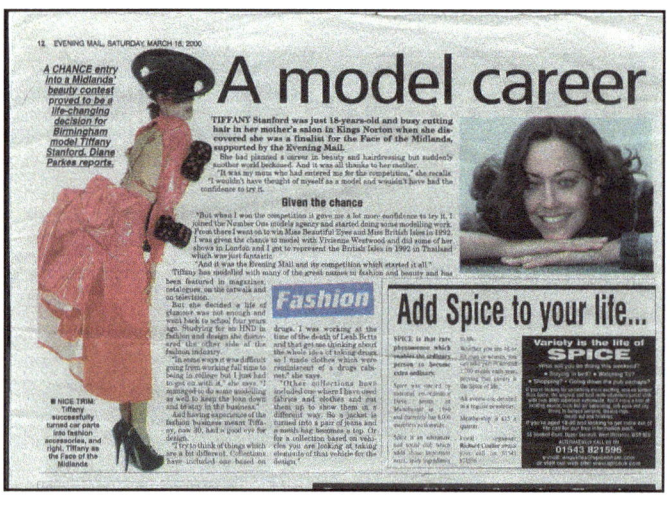

One of my HND fashion designs featured in the Birmingham Evening Mail and based on a car theme.

say no they might be sent home. It's very difficult complaining to an agency as they don't want to lose a client either, so most of the time an agency 'won't want to rock the boat' and are on their client's side.

Equity is a union for actors. Everyone who pays the yearly fee to join will work to a set of rules governed by Equity. This union was set up by a group of performers in 1930 and has been going ever since from strength to strength and recently a division was opened for models who were working at London Fashion Week to make sure that there is a basic salary, no one under the age of 16 can work on the shows and that the models have an employment contract. Basically, it outlines that a model can't be expected to start work at 4am, do shows until 5pm with no food or drink, without sitting down because "the clothes may crease". Maybe this will be the beginning of something big to protect us models?

STYLIST/STYLING

A stylist, fashion stylist or celebrity stylist generally helps to coordinate, put together and have ideas on how all the clothes, props and styling should look. They make sure all the jewellery, clothing, props and accessories look as they should for the photo shoot or show.

They have an important role as the models need to look alluring and perfect, highlighting the trend of the season, whilst having to be different at the same time.

Fashion stylists generally make a person look and feel beautiful and make the clothes stand out; they are able to achieve this through an understanding of the latest trends, colour theory and lighting. It can be a challenging and stressful job, as they have to be able to achieve innovative, exciting fashion looks for their clients, either on a personal level (celebrities, business people) or for a company and they really have to be one step ahead. A good stylist is treasured, as they can make their client shine by choosing the correct clothing and accessories that will highlight the best features of the client, and they will also work with the best hairdressers and make-up artists.

There are different stylists who can be involved in a one-on-one service. These are a few below:

Personal shoppers – they will help you to understand your body shape and what suits you. They accompany you on a shopping trip giving you advice on where and what to buy, how to mix and match clothes, use accessories and

Do You Wannabe a Model?

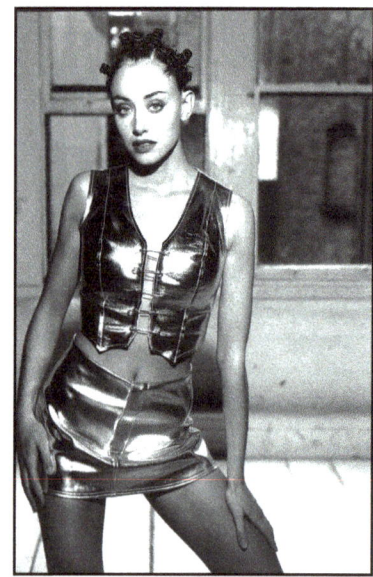

An outfit Tiffany wore out clubbing – oh the good old days.

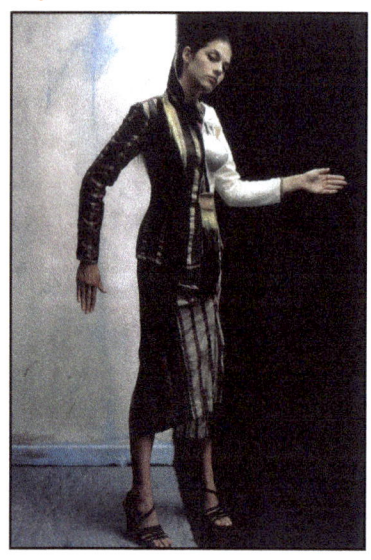

One of Tiffany's designs from the Saville Row capsule collection for her degree at Northampton University. Tiffany won best design originality for the collection.

generally they make you feel a lot more confident about yourself and your wardrobe.

Colour consultant – Most people generally wear colours that THEY think they suit. Black is chosen as it's generally slimming and flattering but colour consultants will help you to understand and wear colours that are most flattering for your skin, eye and hair colour. They will also teach you to combine different shades that work well together. By wearing the right colours you will look brighter and more alive.

Image consultant – they will help you look at your body shape and your skin colour as this generally dictates what clothes look the best on you. As the average size woman in the UK is a 14 you need to understand how to accentuate good points and learn to disguise problem areas. No matter what your size or shape they will help you achieve a look that is best for you and your body frame.

Tiffany is a fully trained image consultant. As she has styled on many fashion photo shoots, hair salons and catwalk shows here are some of her fashion tips:

- **Dress for your shape** – there is nothing worse than people wearing clothes that are too small and with lumps and bumps hanging out! Dress for your shape, not for a trend, and wear the correct size. Then you can feel really happy about yourself.

- **Dress it up** – accessories are such a great way to change the look of any outfit. Use belts, jewellery, gloves and bags. It will totally change the outfit.

- **Underwear tips** – wear the correct size bra by getting yourself professionally measured. Underwear gives you a silhouette and makes sure everything stays in place. If you need a little help holding things in, get Spandex underwear. They are just brilliant!!

- **Style is ageless** – don't feel that because of your age you have to dress a certain way. Just dress for your shape.

- **Break the rules** – don't stick to too many rules with colour. Experiment! I know black can be slimming but be brave and wear colours. If wearing colours together, ensure they are of the same tone. Colour can reflect you and your personality!

- **Customise your wardrobe** – try different things out, experiment with your clothes and create your own look. Make sure you own a well fitted pair of jeans. They can be a saviour.

- **Co-ordinate outfits** – hang pieces of clothes that work well together and dress to your strengths.

- **Fashion care** – take good care of your clothes. Wash them correctly, according to the labels. Maybe redye your faded clothes and recycle where possible. Charity shops have some fantastic bargains, if you're good at putting items together.

- **Work your wardrobe** – separate your wardrobe into three sections: everyday, workwear and glamour. Try and mix and match all three.

- **Experiment** – don't just try and follow current fashion

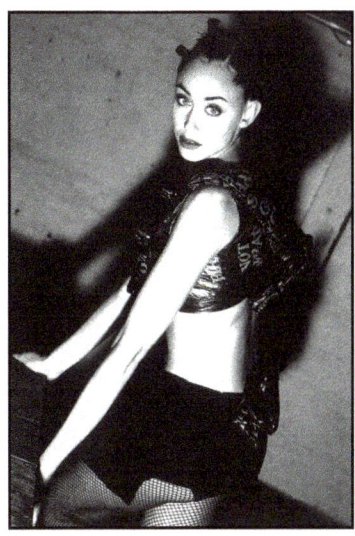

A wild outfit that Tiffany made to go clubbing in – yes it is a bin bag as a top!

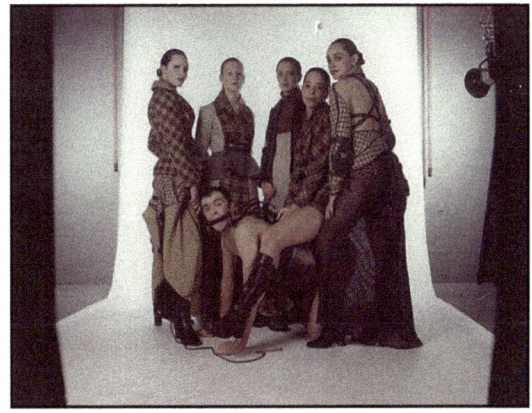

Tiffany on the right wearing the design she created for Miss Great Britain's national costume 98 worn by Lelanie Dowling in the Miss Universe pageant.

trends as they change every six months and can get expensive to follow. Add colour to an outfit – e.g. use a pink scarf or stilettos to brighten up a black outfit.

Accessory advice

Belts will finish off an outfit; they can also enhance your waistline.

Jewellery; too much can ruin an outfit, but none at all can look too understated.

Handbags are my favourite accessory. Choose a small sturdy one for everyday use that will go with everything. Then buy small, coloured bags to match different outfits.

Scarves can liven up and enhance an outfit and can also change a daytime look to an evening.

Sunglasses really should suit the shape of your face and if you wear prescription glasses make sure your sunglasses are too.

Gloves aren't just for celebrities! They can make an outfit look beautiful, really classy and glamorous.

Fashion trends

Fashion changes every six months and can really be very expensive to try and keep up with. Try not to follow all the latest trends. Be different and create your own style that suits you, your personality and body shape.

Below are some sites you can view and have fun looking at for any fashion ideas:

www.elle.com, www.style.com, www.refinery29.com, www.vogue.co.uk, www.fashiontrendlatest.com

SPECIALISED UNDERWEAR

Tights

At some point in our lives, whether 18 or 80, we all suffer from tired aching legs. This can happen to any one of us, even if we keep active.

Some people also suffer from varicose veins which can be unsightly and uncomfortable. These can be caused by your job i.e. standing for long periods of time. During long periods of inactivity, blood can pool in the veins of the legs, which can cause a feeling of heaviness and sometimes causes swollen ankles. If these symptoms persist, this can lead to varicose veins. Prevention

Specialised Underwear

is better than cure and support tights are the answer. They apply a gentle pressure all over the leg and this gives a massaging effect, thus ensuring a healthy circulation through the leg. If you are going to use support tights with a denier 14 or higher, we suggest you seek medical advice before you use them for the first time.

Benefits of wearing support tights

- improves circulation.
- conceals varicose veins.
- can be a prevention to costly surgery.
- can help prevent occurrence after surgery.

Helpful tips to prevent tired legs

1. Don't sit for long periods of time with your legs crossed.
2. Avoid clothing that restricts the circulation of the blood in your legs.
3. Exercise your legs and ankles as much as possible.
4. Whenever possible, elevate and rest your legs.

Simple exercises

- Sitting or lying on the floor, flex the foot.
- Rotate the ankles.

Spanx

Spanx is a company which makes support underwear, endorsed by a lot of celebrities such as Gwyneth Paltrow and Sarah Jessica Parker. They make a range of products to make women more confident about their figures as the underwear improves the lines of the body. Spanx underwear has been designed to deal with a multitude of common body problems that many woman notice as they get older or put on weight. Spanx products are seamless to add to comfort, are thin, so they don't add bulk, and they are stretchy. They have no large uncomfortable bands, like other support products, that hold in the legs or the tummy so tight that other problems arise in other areas. Spanx's variety of products are available in black, white and nude and can be purchased in many department stores and from www.magicknickers.com.

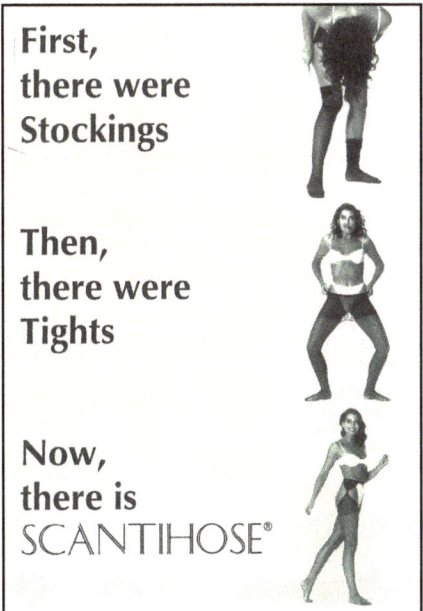

Jeanne in Scantihose advert.

HAIRDRESSING

Tiffany trained for five years to be a professional hairdresser. This is her advice. Our hair is unique, and differs depending on our ethnic origin. Melanin is the hair pigment which gives the hair its colour.

The hair shaft can be easily damaged and can cause split ends (Trichoptilosis). There are many reasons why split ends occur: excessive use of heating tools, straighteners and hairdryers, using the wrong hair shampoos, too many styling products, and bad brushes and combs.

So to avoid causing your hair to get too many split ends and to look after your hair on a daily basis we recommend that you use good hair tools and in the correct way as follows:

Wide Tooth detangling comb – this is a must if you have medium to long hair. It's great for detangling (on wet or dry hair), combing through conditioners, or if you chemically process your hair. Be gentle and always start from the bottom of your hair and work your way up to the roots.

Tail Combs – these are great for backcombing the hair (try not to over backcomb as this can cause knots), sectioning the hair ready for styling and to create a zigzag effect in your hair parting. To backcomb your hair take small sections at the top of your head and start at the roots.

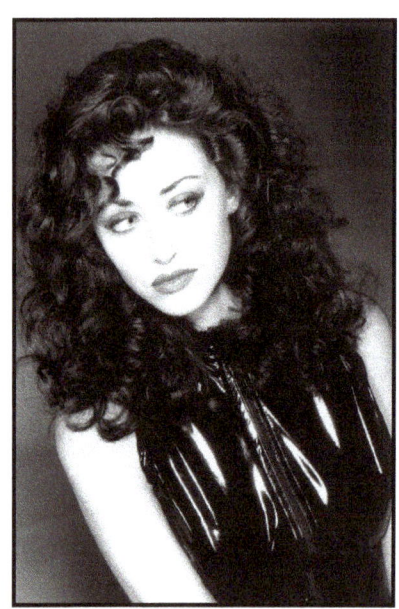

Tiffany hair modelling.

Try and choose a brush that you are comfortable using and is best for your hair. Below are some possible options:

Round hair brush – you can roll hair over or under the brush, so these are generally used to give curl and definition to hairstyles. The smaller the brush the tighter the curl, so for longer hair use a larger round brush, which is generally used to curl the ends of the hair.

Vent hair brush – these have holes in the middle which let air pass through the brush allowing for faster blow-drying and can also boost volume to the hair.

Paddle hair brush – for straightening medium to long hair, this brush smoothes the hair. It is also better for hair that hasn't been layered too much.

Remember to clean your combs and brushes regularly with warm water and liquid soap, and leave to air dry.

The best and easiest way to look after your hair, and the only way to remove split ends as often as possible and continue to do so as part of any beauty regime, is to get your hair cut regularly, usually about every 6-8 weeks. A good haircut/style can also change the look of your hair, bringing about a good change in your appearance. Adequate hair care can make your hair feel healthy, look different and leave it easier to manage (as described above).

Different hairstyles suit the various shaped faces. A useful way to find out what your face shape is, is to look into a mirror and draw with a lip liner onto the mirror around your face and examine the result. www.ukhairdressers.com features different face shapes and shows a large range of different styles available to suit your face shape i.e. layered hair cuts, various short and long hair cuts.

We can be influenced with our style by our favourite pop stars or celebrities, and the fashion industry with both hair and clothes can be very fickle. These things change very quickly, so try to remember to choose a style that will suit you! Other quick ways to change your appearance are to use some hair pieces, braid extensions or to buy a wig. They can allow for a dramatic style change and add length and thickness to your hair. Again, I would highly recommend getting a professional salon to insert the braid/extensions for you and to buy a wig that will suit your face shape.

It is important to go to a reputable hair salon in the UK where the staff are qualified to do your hair and to look after it well. You can look online for a variety of good salons. There is a huge amount of hair salons to select from, ranging from trendy salons like Toni and Guy, to more local salons in your home town. The choice is yours.

Hairdressing prices will vary depending on where you go, but let's say for a simple cut and blow dry, you can expect to pay around £20.00. I suggest that you check the costs when you book your hair appointment.

Another quick way to change your appearance is by changing the colour of your hair. Most of the hair colouring products are user friendly and smell a lot less chemical than they used to. I recommend that hair colouring is done by a professional qualified hairdresser.

Remember, you must always have a skin test 24-48 hours before ever applying hair dye to see if you are allergic to the chemicals in the mixture. This must be done at a salon and should be done even if you are doing the treatment yourself at home.

There are a few different types of hair colouring available.

Permanent colouring enriches the natural hair tones and is applied to dry hair. It can colour grey hair and can darken or lighten your usual hair colour by up to two shades. The staying power is better than other methods as it grows out of the hair with your natural hair growth and therefore the hair roots will need to be redyed every four to six weeks.

Semi-permanent colouring also enriches the natural hair colour by a shade darker. These dyes will wash out or fade after about 4-6 weeks. The colour should be applied to wet hair and does not have a regrowth. It generally conditions the hair without leaving it dry.

Temporary colouring is a wash-in dye that is applied to wet hair and only usually lasts for a few washes. It is the kindest to the hair as it doesn't contain many strong chemicals.

Bleaching/highlights are when peroxide is applied to the hair either via a hair cap or using tin foil. It strips away the hair melanin to achieve various shades of blonde depending on your original hair colour. This will also grow out with your hair, leaving darker roots. It will need to be re-done every four to six weeks.

Other hair techniques that can change your appearance are perming/curling/relaxing your hair, either permanently or not. The permanent wave is achieved by winding the hair around different sized perm curlers and set by using certain chemicals and this will generally last around three months depending on how often the hair is cut. A permanent wave can help with the thickness of the hair, giving it more bounce if the hair is fine.

Relaxing is done on afro-caribbean hair and involves the use of the chemical sodium hydroxide which, when smoothed on to the hair in sections, makes the hair straight. For more information on it and products to use, go to: www.blackhairinformation.com

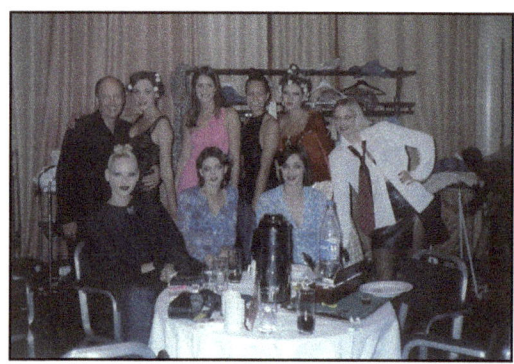

Left back: Trevor Sorbie and Tiffany.

Curling your hair with rollers, tongs or straighteners again gives the hair an immediately different look and as long as it is done correctly, using the correct hair styling products, it won't be too damaging to the hair. Personally, I prefer to use the ceramic straighteners (GHDs), which are generally kinder to the hair, and perhaps using a heat protectant spray will also help to protect your hair, especially if you dry and straighten your hair every day. Also, try to use the hairdryer on a lower heat so as not to over dry your hair.

Some different hair types:

Fine hair – blondes are most likely to have fine hair. As it is the thinnest, try volumising hair products, gentle shampoo and a lightweight conditioner on the ends.

Medium hair – this is the most common hair type. It is soft, manageable and is considered 'normal' hair. Most shampoos and conditioners will suit it.

Coarse hair – Rough, wiry, heavy, strong and dry, it is harder to manage and will need a good strong conditioner.

Here are two ways to find out what your hair type is:

- How long does it take for your hair to dry naturally? If it's less than an hour then your hair is fine. Your hair is thick if it takes more than an hour to dry.
- Put your hair in a ponytail, put your thumb and fore finger round it, if the circle is ten pence size or less it is fine hair. It is thick if the circle is a fifty pence piece or more, while any thing in between is medium.

Dry hair – this is due to inactive oil glands in the scalp which lacks moisture. This can be a natural condition and may be aggravated by exposure to the sun, using harsh shampoos or any chemical treatments. Dry hair can look dull and have split ends. Use a mild or herbal shampoo at least three times a week with a good conditioner.

Oily hair – this is due to excessive secretion of oil from glands. Oily hair needs to be washed daily. PH levels on the scalp can be controlled by using herbal shampoos. A conditioner may not need to be used: it depends on how oily the hair is.

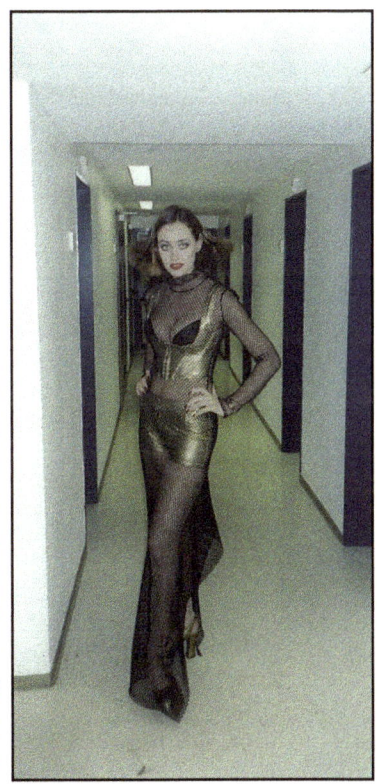

Tiffany modelling for Trevor Sorbie hair show. What an outfit!

Do You Wannabe a Model?

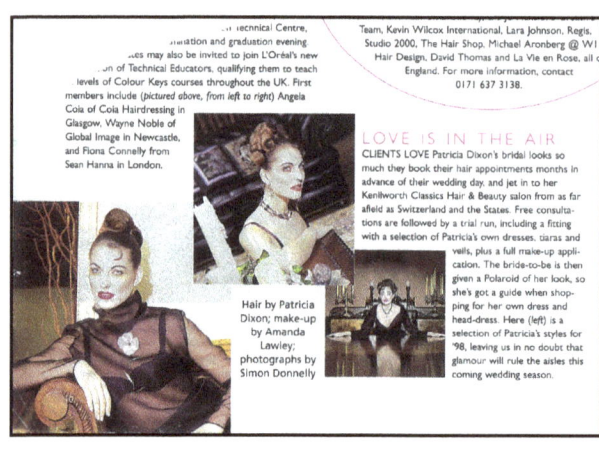

Tiffany and Jeanne appearing in a magazine together. Courtesy of Pat Dixon Hair.

Normal hair – usually shiny, well balanced and the most ideal hair type. Look after it well on a regular basis to maintain the health and shine.

Combination hair – this means a greasy scalp and dry ends. The ends are split and lighter in colour than the root.

To find out what type of hair you have follow these instructions:

The day after washing, rub a tissue on the scalp. If it gets an oil blot then you have normal hair. If there is nothing on the tissue then your hair is dry. If the hair strands stick to each other due to grease then you have oily hair.

Styling products:

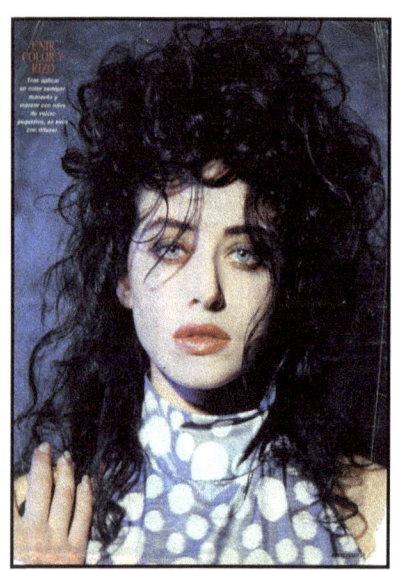

Tiffany hair modelling.

These can offer an immediate effect or change while experimenting with latest styles. There are several products to help you to manage hair: gels, mousses, waxes, serums, sprays and creams. They can transform your hair from frizzy to flat, coarse to soft, and thin to thick. Find out which one is best to use for your hair type. All the products mentioned are soft to touch and can be easily removed from the hair as long as they are applied correctly, as instructed. Whilst using the products and styling your hair, it is recommended to use a low heat on your hairdryer to prevent too much damage.

While these modern hairstyle products and treatments can offer you a stylish new look, the consequences should not be over-

HAIRDRESSING

looked. You must always take great and special care of your hair (whatever your origin) by using the right hair products and by frequently going to the right professional hair salon.

Some helpful hair tips:

Big Bouncy Curls – to create big curls, section your hair and using your GHD irons vertically start at the base of the head at the roots and slowly slide half way down, then twist the irons and pull the hair through, continuing to twist.

Messy Bun – decide where you want the bun to be and secure your ponytail with a hair bobble. Using a small comb roughly backcomb the ponytail. Grabbing sections of the ponytail loop it and pin the hair to create a rough doughnut shape. Continue until you are happy with your bun.

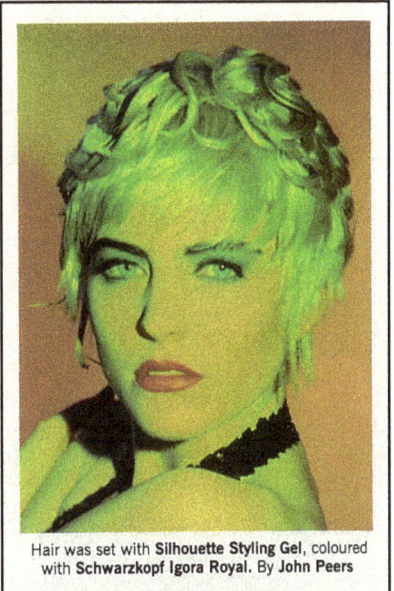

Hair was set with **Silhouette Styling Gel**, coloured with **Schwarzkopf Igora Royal**. By **John Peers**

Jeanne in a hair magazine modelling a wig.

French Pleat – brush all your hair back and gather to one side. At the centre back of the head create a line of grips to hold the hair in place. Pull the hair to the opposite side making sure the hair is smooth. With your hand twist the hair towards the grips to create a roll shape and then tuck in any remainder hair and all along the roll secure with the grips and pins.

Volume – start below the crown and section the hair. From the bottom hold a section of hair up vertically and start to backcomb it from the mid-lengths to the roots. Work your way up through the sections and repeat until you get the volume you want. Remember to backcomb the underside so that it isn't too obvious.

SKIN THROUGHOUT THE YEARS

All women age differently and genes generally determine how well our skin ages. However you can help yourself by following these simple rules:

1. Drink plenty of water (recommended amount is two litres a day).
2. Stay out of the sun.
3. Avoid smoking.

Do You Wannabe a Model?

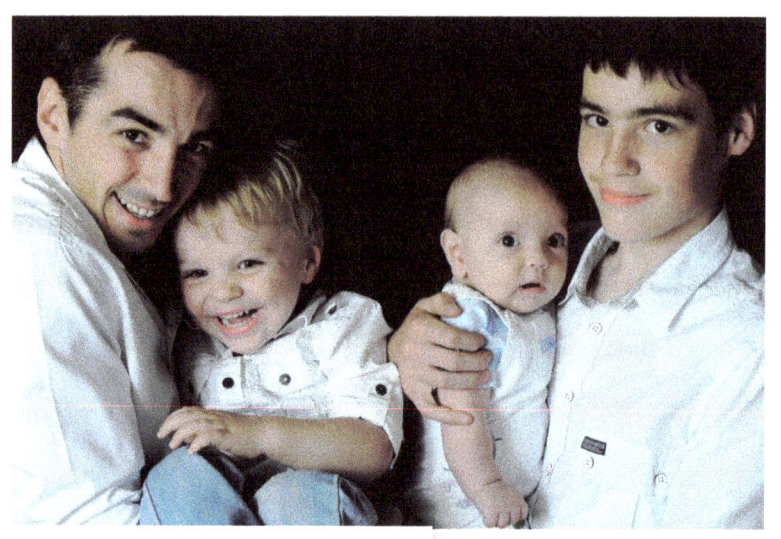

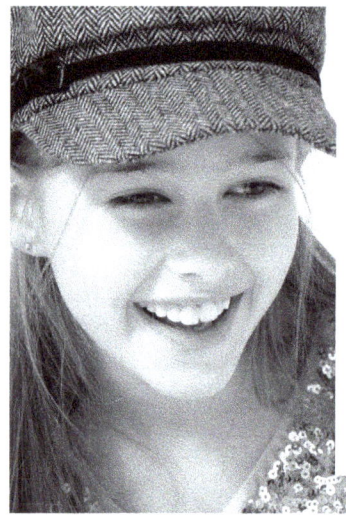

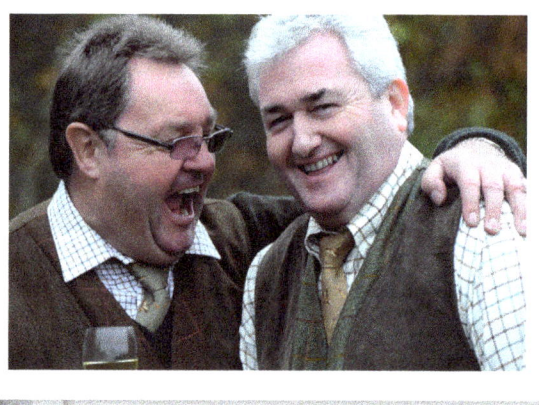

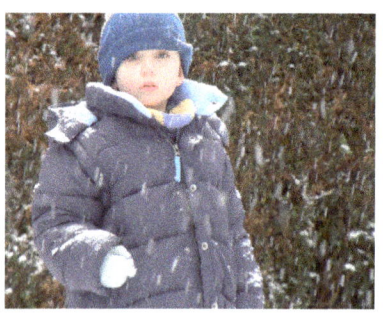

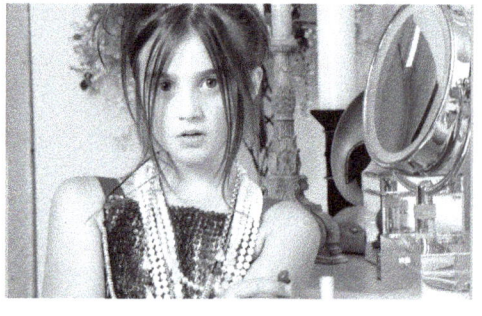

Jeanne's Professional Photography

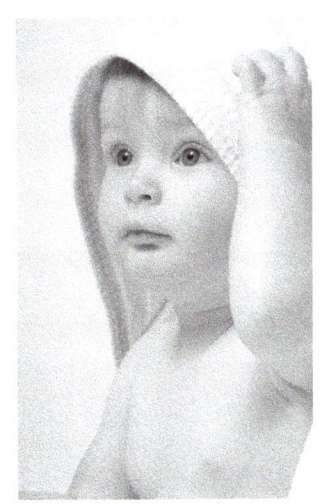
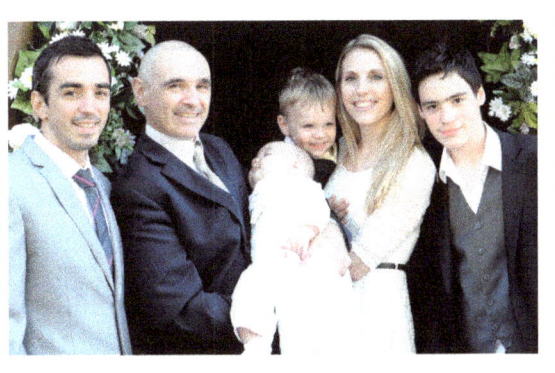
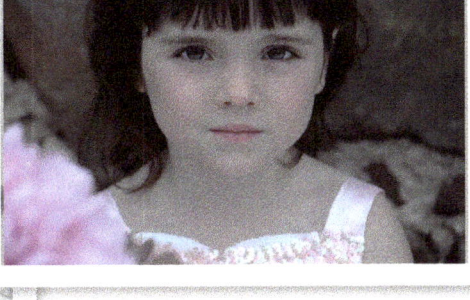
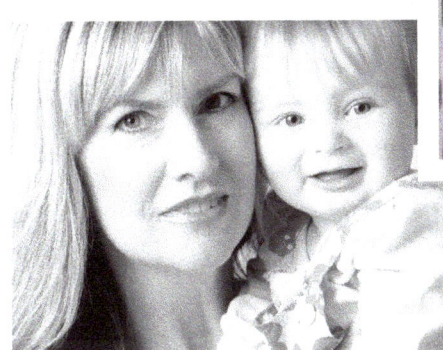

A selection of Jeanne's professional photography.
www.jeannefrithphotography.co.uk

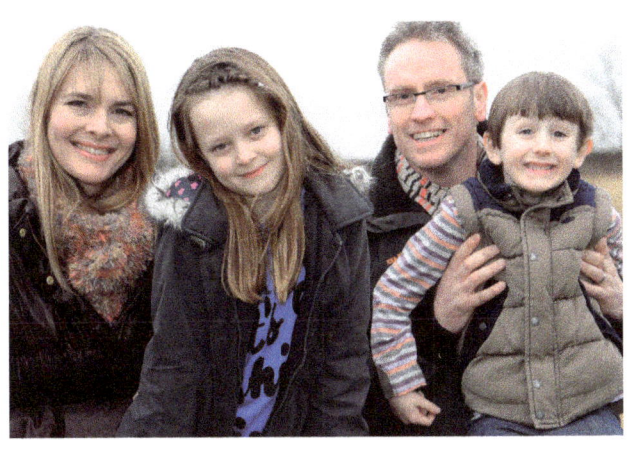

Teen Years

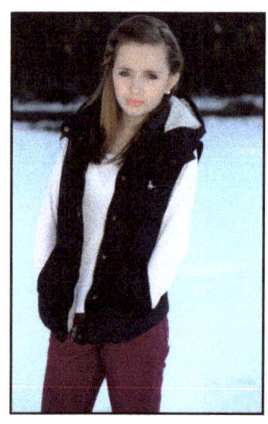

In your teen years you may be constantly battling against blemishes and acne. This can be linked to your menstrual cycle but maybe you are just an unlucky teenager. Jeanne had always had fairly good skin and then, in her mid 20s (fairly old), she started to suffer from very bad acne all over her face. Normally her blemishes would be in her T-zone (across the forehead and down the nose and chin) and would be related to her periods. For no reason her skin got very painful big spots (boils) and when they were squeezed nothing came out. It can be very embarrassing having acne of the face as a photographic model. A make-up artist recommended to Jeanne on a photo shoot a product called *Ketsugo*. It can be bought from most high street chemists like Superdrug and Boots and costs around £12.00. It was great for Jeanne and levelled out her pH balance which cleared her skin. You can also try Wannabe Workshops' suggested beauty products from Arbonne. Go to www.wannabeworkshops.com and follow the link to Arbonne. The FC5 is brilliant for young skin and the conditioning oil at £12.00 is perfect for that problem spot.

If you do suffer from acne try not to always wear make-up, give your skin the chance to breath. When you do wear make-up, make sure you use a light foundation and a concealer rather than any heavy foundation. Follow a skin care regime twice a day and use products to suit your skin type.

Top tips for beautiful skin!

Never sleep with your make-up on. If you are too tired to cleanse, tone and moisturise, take make-up off with face wipes. Don't do this too often but every now and again is fine.

The 20s

These really are the best years for your skin. You should have a beauty regime in place which you do regularly. Don't forget when applying moisturiser to apply it to your face and neck, hands and around the eye area. Also at this age do not over-pluck your eyebrows as when you get older they thin out and you don't want to end up without any by the time you are 40.

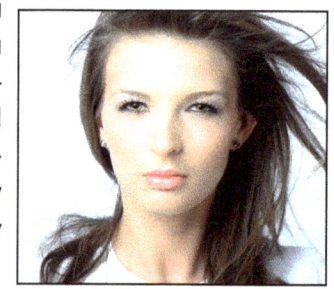

The 30s

At this age you may start to notice your skin is drier and fine lines maybe more visible around the eyes, lips and forehead. A serum under your moisturiser should be added to your regular beauty regime and a primer can be used before applying a foundation. This fills the fine lines and avoids the foundation from getting the 'cracking' look. A great product is Arbonne primer (www.wannabeworkshops.com). This gives a radiance boost and revives the skin for a softer, smoother looking complexion. You will find that most brands do sell a version of this so see if people have any samples that you try and find one that best suits you and your skin. At this age use a sunscreen or buy a moisturiser with a SPF. A good exfoliator should be used once a week. Having facials, if you can afford it, are not only beneficial but also very relaxing if you are now juggling a career as well as a family life. A good facial will cost around £35.

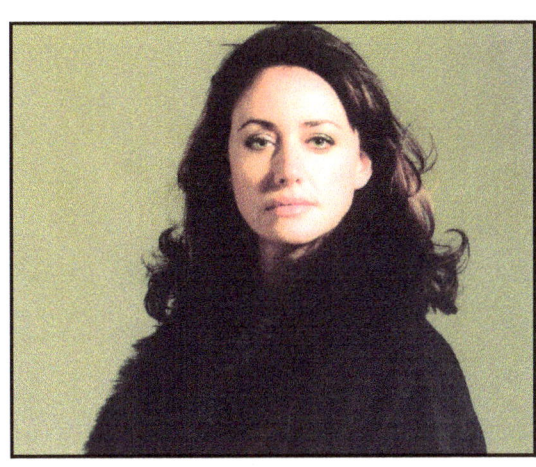

Skin in the 30s. Tiffany's last test shoot aged 34 – still got it.

The 40s +

What suited your skin in your 20s is not suitable now. You should be using a richer moisturiser, a serum and a night cream as well as using an eye cream. Use masks and exfoliators regularly. Your skin will be much drier and will not retain moisture as well as it used to. Shop around when buying products. Try different brands until you find one that suits your skin type and your purse. Be aware that more expensive does not always mean better. We are all different and what suits you may not suit others, so it is a case of trial and error. Arbonne do an excellent anti-ageing range (check out www.wannabeworkshops.com).

Facials cost around £35 from a good reputable beauty salon. They last approximately an hour and there are different types available from anti-ageing, to aromatherapy. It is up to you what you choose to have and also what you want to achieve from the treatment.

SKIN TYPES

There are five different skin types. A good test to find out your skin type is: When you wake up in the morning, before doing anything, wipe your face with a tissue. Oily skin will leave an oily residue. Normal skin will leave no oil and will not feel dry and scratchy. Dry skin, even first thing in the morning, will be dry. Most people have combination skin and you will get a mixture of dryness and oily patches. With sensitive skin you will learn with trial and error. If you use a product and you feel a burning and itchy feeling, stop using it immediately. Consult a doctor if problem persists.

Oily skin – this skin type needs maximum care, as it is prone to acne, pimples and breakouts. Special care is needed so use formulated washes. It is best to use an astringent and when choosing moisturisers use water-based ones. Gel creams and lotions are good for oily skin. A mild scrub should be used to remove blackheads and dead skin cells.

Normal skin – if you have normal skin you are one of the lucky ones. This skin type just requires a normal cleansing, toning and moisturising regime. Once a fortnight, a face pack for normal skin types could be applied to keep the skin fresh looking.

Combination skin – this is where your face has a mixture of dry and oily patches. The dry areas are normally found on the cheeks and the oily areas are normally found in what is called the T-zone, across the forehead, down the nose and in the crease of the chin. Caring for combination skin requires a mild cleanser, and use of an astringent on the oily parts of the face. When applying moisturiser, concentrate on the dry areas. Combination skin is the most common skin type.

Dry skin – dry skin has a thin texture and can look visibly dry when in its natural state. It can also have red patches. This type of skin, like oily skin, needs special care. It requires face washes and creams for dry skin. Always apply a good night cream before going to bed. An advantage of having dry skin is it hardly ever has a breakout of spots and pimples.

Sensitive skin – this skin can be sensitive to dirt, dust, sun and most creams, soap and lotions. It can get itchy and have patches of redness. It will break out easily. You have to be very careful. You should only use mild skin products, lotions, creams and moisturisers which have been especially designed for sensitive skin. Never use any perfumed products. Always inform a make-up artist that you have sensitive skin.

Skin Types

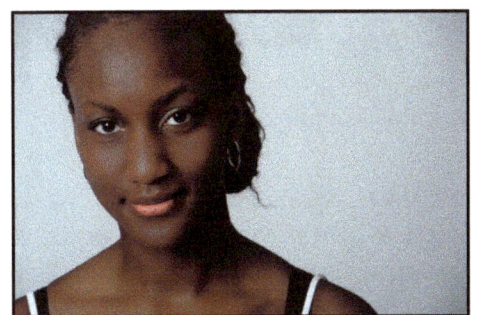

Ethnic skin tone – afro-caribbean skin has more sebaceous glands so can be oilier. This helps to protect against the process of ageing – although the skin can still be dry. Skin has four types: combination, oily, dry and normal. (See previous notes.)

CLEANSING, TONING AND MOISTURISING

Men, women and young adults should all cleanse, tone and moisturise on a daily basis and exfoliate the skin (maybe use an Arbonne product) at least once a week which will get rid of dead skin cells. Your face is the most constantly exposed feature of the body to the environment. Your skin is the organ that protects everything within the body so it is essential to look after it. An early start to taking care of the face can prevent and deter problems of the skin such as acne, wrinkles and other annoying skin ailments. This five minute daily routine will not only keep the epidermis (surface layer of skin) supple and healthy, but help keep the deeper dermis tissue and muscles toned and healthy.

Cleansing instructions: Moisten a flannel with warm water. With both hands start at the neck and moisten the neck and face upward and outward with circular motions. This is essential to remove the dead skin cells. Using a 10p sized portion of facial cleanser, dab a small amount on either side of the Adam's apple, the chin, both sides of the lower jaw, each cheek, each side of the nose, each eyelid, each temple and a few dabs across the forehead. With the finger tips work in small circular motions, upward and outward starting at the neck. Work up the neck and face methodically. When completed, moisten the flannel again with warm water and rinse off the cleanser thoroughly.

> ### JEANNE'S TOP TIPS
>
> EXERCISE REGULARLY – A GOOD TIP IS TO EXERCISE 5 TIMES DURING THE WEEK AND HAVE THE WEEKEND OFF. IF WORK AND FAMILY LIFE ALLOW, MY EXERCISE ROUTINE LOOKS LIKE THIS: MONDAY – A 3-MILE RUN AND AN HOUR OF YOGA; TUESDAY – A 3-MILE RUN AND A 30-MIN WALK; WEDNESDAY – AN HOUR'S ZUMBA CLASS AND 30-MIN WALK; THURSDAY – A BODY BALANCE CLASS AND A 30-MIN WALK; FRIDAY – A 2-MILE RUN. THE WEEKENDS I HAVE OFF WITH NO GUILT! VARYING THE EXERCISE IS THE KEY TO MAINTAINING IT SO YOU DON'T GET BORED!

Toning: Using toner or aftershave, cover the cleansed surface of the neck and face. If it makes it easier, moisten a piece of cotton wool with the toner or aftershave. Rub the solution on the neck and face in the same upward and outward motions used for cleansing.

Exfoliating: Using a gentle product like Neutrogena, exfoliate your skin at least once a week. Wash your face with warm water then using a pea size amount of the product do circular movements with your fingertips around your neck and face, avoiding your eye area, and then wash off with warm water.

Moisturising: Put small drops of moisturiser on each side of the neck, the chin, each side of the lower jaw, each cheek, each side of the nose, each eyelid, each temple and about three blobs across the forehead. Smooth the moisturiser all over the neck and face in circular motions upward and outward as before.

There are two different types of moisturisers. A day moisturiser and a night moisturiser. There are benefits to both. A day moisturiser should have an SPF 15 or higher, but no less, and always use an anti-ageing one when you are in your 30s. This protects the face against harmful sunrays. A night moisturiser must only be used at night-time when you are sleeping as it replenishes the skin and also intensely hydrates the skin, but night moisturisers are far too heavy for daytime use.

There are facial wipes which are good for convenience if you are out and about. They are pre-moistened and some are oil free. They instantly dissolve all traces of dirt, oil and make-up deep down to the pores. They are readily available at any pharmacy or most supermarkets.

There are many good cleansers, toners and moisturisers sold by the big brands including Arbonne, Clarins, Elemis, Clinque, Elizabeth Arden No 7, No17, Nivea, and Oil of Olay. They all come in different price brackets too, so try one that is in your price range and work from there. Many companies do trial sizes so you don't have to spend huge amounts of money to find out what suits you.

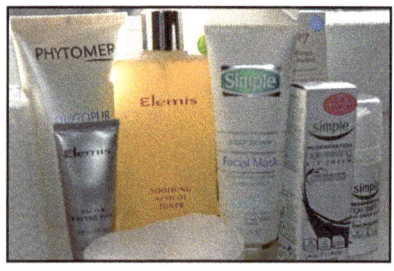

Don't be fooled into thinking the most expensive will be the best for your skin. Many different brands contain the same ingredients so you may just be paying for the name of the brand. Look at the labels to see which one claims to suit your skin type. Ask for samples, if possible, to trial, and find a range of products to suit you. Discontinue using any product that causes a bad reaction.

ANTI-AGEING PRODUCTS

> **TIFFANY'S TOP TIPS**
>
> ENJOY ALL YOUR EXPERIENCES AND THE JOBS YOU DO – LIFE GOES QUICKLY.

Anti–ageing products are generally marketed towards women who are of a certain age. They are predominantly moisturiser-based skincare products and are used as part of your daily skincare routine. They promise to tighten any skin sagging, reduce visible wrinkles, expression lines, and other environmentally related conditions of the skin.

Some anti-ageing products may also have other ingredients added: retinol (this helps reduce fine lines), sunscreens, antioxidants (to protect skin cells), vitamin C. The effects of the products' ingredients can depend on how concentrated it is, how regularly it is used and how old the user is.

SPF

This is the Sun Protection Factor displayed on sunscreen labels, face moisturisers and in foundations. It can range from 2-50 + and refers to the products' ability to block out the sun's harmful rays during the day. The sunrays are there even on cloudy days. 80% of the sun's ultraviolet rays can pass through the clouds, and these are known as UVB and UVA. UVA are the rays that penetrate deeper into the skin and are the culprits in premature ageing and wrinkling of the skin. This is why it is important to start using skin products with an SPF to prevent your skin ageing prematurely. You are never too young to start and my advice is to always use a high SPF whilst out in the sun. Although the sun is wonderful, it is very ageing.

On most occasions a minimum of SPF 15 should be used in your suncream, face moisturiser and foundation. Sun cream should be reapplied throughout the day and use waterproof ones. If you use a sunscreen with an SPF 20 you can stay in the sun 20 times longer than without before burning and so on.

FACE TYPES

The best way to find out what your face shape is, is to look into a mirror and draw with a lip liner or an eyeliner onto the mirror around your face shape and examine the results. The most flattering face shape is an oval. Contouring and highlighting can be used to slightly alter the shape your face appears to be. It will give the illusion of a perfect symmetrical face. You can also enhance or reduce the appearance of certain features.

Contouring and shading plays down flaws and can add depth.

Highlighting enhances good points by reflecting the light to lift features.

Where to shade:

1. **Shade** – under the cheekbones to add definition, create cheekbones where they are not visible and slim down the face.

2. **Shade** – the temples to soften a square face to make a wide forehead appear narrower.

3. **Contour** – the eye to add depth, shading along and slightly above the crease.

4. **Shading** – under the lip will shorten a long nose.

Where to highlight:

1. **Highlight** – on the top of cheekbones to bring them forward and enhance them.

2. **Highlight** – to open up eyes and make them bigger, highlight on the arch of the eyebrow and on the inner corner of the eye.

3. **Highlight** – under the outer corners of the eyes to give the eyes an instant lift and waken up tired eyes.

4. **Highlight** – just above the top lip along the bow and under the outer edges to give lips a fuller shape.

When to contour and highlight:

Highlight – If you are trying to disguise a wide nose. Highlight the bridge of the nose, vertically down the centre then shade down either side of the nostril. Add highlight on the cheeks directly to the edge of the nostrils.

Square face – A square face has a strong squared jawline and a broad forehead. The width and length are in proportion but the corners are more angular. If contouring, the main areas are the centre of the forehead and down the centre of the nose. Blusher can be brushed vertically on either side to soften the width.

Long face – This shape face is longer than it is wide. The forehead, cheekbones and jaw line are all one width. To disguise a long face, contour on the chin and hair line. Highlight on top of the cheekbones and apply a blusher horizontally.

Oval face – This shape face is considered to be the perfect shape because it is completely balanced in proportions. The angles of the face are perfect for applying make-up. The forehead is wider than the chin and the cheekbones are strong and prominent. This face shape suits all styles of make-up.

Heart shape – This shape face is similar to the oval as the forehead is wide but then it curves down to the chin. The chin can be softened with highlighting and shading, and the forehead can have shading at the temples to make the forehead appear narrower. Applying blusher on the apples of the cheeks will soften the overall shape.

Round shape – This shape face appears youthful. The length and width are in good proportion and there are no angles. The cheekbones are hidden by wide cheeks. Use contouring and highlighting to enhance the appearance of a round face and bring out the angles and the cheekbones. Apply blusher on the underside of the cheekbones at a slant.

> **JEANNE'S TOP TIPS**
>
> DRY BODY BRUSH – DO THIS BEFORE A SHOWER OR BATH. START FROM YOUR LEGS AND WORK UP. WORK AREAS SUCH AS THE BOTTOM AND THE THIGHS. ALWAYS BRUSH TOWARDS THE HEART. THIS IS EXCELLENT FOR REDUCING CELLULITE.

HOW TO APPLY MAKE-UP TO ETHNIC SKIN TONE

The key to success when applying make-up is to choose deep, bold colours. These will give the skin a wonderful glow.

1. Choose a foundation that matches your skin tone. Mixing different shades is a good way to achieve this. Apply the foundation with a damp sponge or brush making sure you blend along the jawline and hairline.

2. Set with a light dusting of translucent loose powder.

3. Sweep a dark blackcurrant eyeshadow over the eyelid. A good tip is to apply some loose powder under the eyes, then if any eyeshadow is dropped onto the face it can be swept away with the loose powder and it does not ruin the previously applied foundation.

4. Apply a dark charcoal eyeshadow in the crease of the eyelid.

5. Use the same dark charcoal eyeshadow on an eyeliner brush and work some under the lower lashes.

6. Finish the eyes with two coats of black mascara.

7. Use a tawny brown shade of blusher to complement the skin colour. Dust

over the cheekbones working towards the hairline if trying to create a more defined look. Dust the apple of the cheeks if trying to achieve a more youthful look.

8. Try to choose a lip colour either the same colour or tone as the blusher as this will give a streamline look from the lips up the face. Apply a lip liner, always following the lip line, then colour in the lips. This will act as a base and will hold the lipstick in place for longer. Apply the lipstick or gloss on top of the lip liner.

Useful Websites
www.imanbeauty.com
www.maccosmetics.co.uk
www.kbybeverleyknightcosmetics.com

NINE STEPS TO NATURAL MAKE-UP FOR A CASTING AND DAY MAKE-UP

1. For best results apply make-up using natural lighting (by a window) or, if in a studio, use a lighted make-up mirror.

2. Wash and moisturise your face. Leave a few minutes before applying make-up to ensure a firm foundation.

3. Using a concealer one or two shades lighter than your natural skin tone, cover all blemishes, spots and dark spots. **Yves Saint Laurent Touche Éclat (Radiant Touch)** is great for disguising dark lines under the eyes.

4. Choose a foundation slightly thicker than usual and use one with a minimum SPF 15 as harmful rays can age your skin. This will give a flawless base and cover all blemishes. Blend the foundation from chin to neck, so it's the same colour all the way down.

5. Powder – use lots of it to create a matt finish. As your shoot continues you can powder throughout the day. Places to be aware of are the forehead, crease of the chin and upper top lip. All these will shine if you get hot under the studio lights.

6. Cheeks – blusher can be put on cheekbones to highlight, or under them to create a contoured look. Think about the finished look that you and the photographer are trying to create. Be careful to blend in the blusher and avoid two harsh lines going down the sides of the face.

7. Eyes – put a pale colour all over eye. On the crease of the eyelid put

a darker shade and blend it in. Using the same colour as the darker shade, go under the eye and blend. If using eyeliner, precision is vital. Again, try and remember the look that you are trying to achieve. Don't go too heavy with black eyeliner if you are trying to get a natural beauty shot. Use a highlighter under the eyebrow arch.

> **TIFFANY'S TOP TIPS**
>
> ALWAYS EAT A GOOD HEALTHY BREAKFAST. IT'S THE MOST IMPORTANT MEAL OF THE DAY.

8. Eyelashes – use two or three thin layers of waterproof mascara. Wait till each layer has dried before applying the next one.

9. Lips – make sure there is a slight coverage of foundation on your lips to act as a base. Using a lip liner go round the edge of the lips try and stay on the natural lip line. Use the same colour lipstick or gloss colour in the lips. For extra staying power blot your lips on a tissue and re-apply the lipstick or gloss.

Don't use a shimmery or frosty eyeshadow as this will reflect and appear shiny on the photograph.

Always make sure that your foundation is blended well along the jaw line.

Never use a lip liner that is darker than the lip stick.

Make-up can be found at most highstreet stores such as Boots, Superdrug and Lloyds Chemist. They sell brands such as Rimmel, Barry M and Revlon. Not all of them sell the expensive brands but these can be found at department stores such as Debenhams, House of Fraser and Selfridges, Harvey Nicholls and Harrods, which are excellent for the more specialised brands such as Mac and Bobbi Brown.

MAKE-UP TIPS FOR MATURE SKIN

Mature skin tends to lose its glow and sparkle over the years and make-up is the perfect tool to camouflage this and imitate youthfulness.

When we get older we get fine lines, wrinkles, freckles and age spots. To cover these imperfections people tend to use a heavier foundation. However, thick matt foundations only bring the eye to the fine lines or dryness. There are four main products that are best to use when applying make-up to a more mature skin.

These are:

1. A skin primer – this is applied after your moisturiser and before your foundation. It acts as a base to your foundation. This will hydrate your skin and also gives a flawless finish.

2. A concealer.
3. A light reflecting foundation.
4. An oil-free loose powder.

Method

• When applying your make-up, start with a concealer. Pay particular attention to stubborn spots i.e. cover hyperpigments. A green base can be used to take away any redness caused by high blood pressure or broken capillaries.

• There are special products to use on dark circles around the eye. These are lighter in texture and light reflecting. YSL do Touche Eclat, which many make-up artists use, but many other beauty companies do their own versions and it is always good to try some trials and find which one best suits you and your skin.

• Using a sponge, apply a light reflecting foundation making sure to blend in well around the hair and jawline. A sponge will ensure a flawless coverage. Light reflectors add luminosity to your skin and soften fine lines. For very dry skin, consider using a moisturising foundation to hydrate.

• Dust on a loose powder with a large brush, tapping off any excess before applying to the face. As we get older fine downy hairs appear on the face and any excess powder will cling to the hairs enhancing and highlighting them. Too much powder will also highlight lines on the face, so you need just a small amount to absorb excess oil.

Eyes

The key to applying make-up to the eye area of mature skin is 'less is more'. Work with the eyes' natural shape. Pink and neutrals, like soft browns and sands, work perfectly. Always use a matt eyeshadow as shimmer ones are only going to enhance wrinkles around the eyes. A slightly darker shade can be used in the crease of the eyelid. Cream or gel eyeliners can be used in plums and browns and work well with older skin. To finish off apply two coats of black mascara to the top lashes. As we get older we tend to lose eye lashes which is more noticeable on the bottom lashes.

Blusher

Think of your colouring when you blush naturally and try and use these tones when using a blusher. Again, as you get older, it is advised to use a cream blush as this is more moisturising and better to use in circular motion on the apple of the cheeks rather than following the cheek bones in a harsh line.

Lips

Lip primers are an amazing invention and, like the skin primer, they act as a base for the lip colour to sit on. They hydrate the lips and also act as a barrier – stopping the 'bleeding' effect that some women get. 'Bleeding' is where the lipstick goes into the fine lines around the lips. Avoid using ultra matt shades and use light pinks, nudes, peaches and apricots that give a younger effect. A lipgloss is a better option to go for rather than a matt lipstick. Only use a lip liner if you're applying lipstick and want a dramatic look. To achieve a natural look no lip liner is needed.

EVENING MAKE-UP

1. When applying make-up try and do it with either natural lighting, for example by a large window. Or if indoors in a studio, try and use a make-up mirror with the lights all around.

2. Wash and moisturise your face.

3. Using a concealer one or two shades lighter than your natural skin tone, cover all blemishes, spots and dark spots. YSL Gold pen is great for disguising dark lines under the eyes.

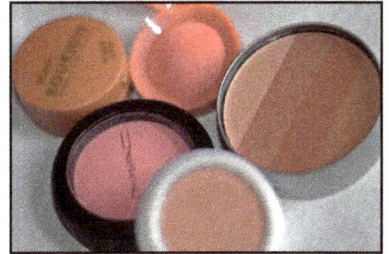

4. Choose a foundation slightly thicker than usual as this will give a flawless base and cover all blemishes. Blend the foundation from chin to neck, so it's the same colour all the way down.

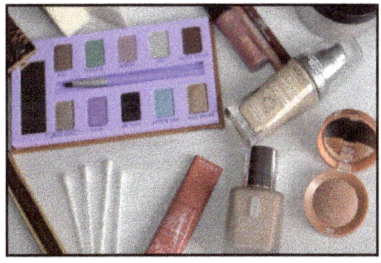

5. Powder – use lots of it: this creates a matt finish. As your shoot continues you can powder throughout the day. Places to be aware of are the forehead, crease of the chin and upper top lip. All these will shine if you get hot under the studio lights.

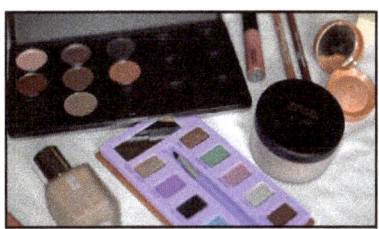

6. Blusher can be put on cheekbones to highlight, or under them to create a contoured look. Think about the finished look that you and the photographer are trying to create. Be careful to blend in the blusher and not have two harsh lines going down the sides of the face.

7. Eyes – put a pale colour all over the eye. On the crease of the eyelid put a darker shade and blend it in. Using the same colour as the darker shade, go under the eye and blend. If using eyeliner, precision is vital. Again try and remember the look that you are trying to achieve. Don't go too heavy with black eyeliner if you are trying to get a natural beauty shot. Use a highlight under the eyebrow arch.

8. Apply two or three thin layers of mascara. Wait till each layer has dried before applying the next one.

9. Lips – make sure there is a slight coverage of foundation on your lips to act as a base. Using a lip liner go round the edge of the lips, trying to stay on the natural lip line. Apply the same colour lipstick or a gloss colour on the lips. For extra staying power blot your lips on a tissue and re-apply the lipstick or gloss.

Some useful make-up websites with various make-up products:

www.arbonneinternational.co.uk

www.maccosmetics.co.uk

www.barrym.com

www.clinique.com

www.loreal.com

www.maybelline.com

www.urbandecay.com

Don't use a shimmery or frosty eyeshadow as this on camera will appear shiny. Always make sure that your foundation is blended well along the jaw line. Never wear black lip liner.

EYES

Close-set eyes
Making them lighter on the corner will widen the appearance of eyes that are too close together. To enhance the effect, extend the outer corners by using dark colours on the outer third of the eye. When applying mascara, brush the outer lashes out. Apply highlighter just below the outer corners of the lower lashes, to draw attention to the outside of the eyelid.

Deep-set eyes
These eyes have recessed sockets and the mobile area of the eyelid is small. Use a light shadow on the lid with a darker colour just above, but do not

put it in the socket line as this will enhance deep set eyes and bring more attention to them. Line both upper and lower lids very close to the lashes.

Wide-set eyes

To make the eyes appear closer together use darker shadow in the inner corners, fading to a lighter colour on the outer corner. Eyebrows should not extend beyond the outer corner of the eye and the inner edges should be kept together. Use eyeliner along the top and bottom lashes. Brush lashes straight up when applying mascara.

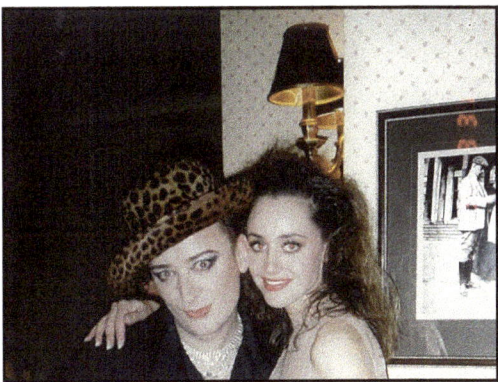

Tiffany and Boy George 1995 at Chuff Chuff.

Small eyes

Apply lighter shades of eyeshadow over the entire eyelid. Start at the lashes and blend towards the brow. Then apply a darker eyeshadow on the outer corner of the eyelid and outer edge of the crease. Use a matt white eyeshade to open up the eye. Line along the top and bottom lash line with a soft brown liner, and use a pale pink pencil inside the lower eyelids. Avoid black eyeliner as it will close the eyes up. Well shaped eyebrows will again open up the eyes. Curl the lashes and coat them with two coats of mascara.

Round eyes

Applying a light coloured eyeshadow on the inner corner of the eyes and fading in to a medium coloured shadow across the middle of the lid will elongate round eyes and make them appear more almond shape. Then use a dark colour on the outer third of the eye and extend it beyond the outer corner, blending downwards along the lower lash line. Line along the top and bottom lashes, flicking the line slightly from the outer corner on the top lid. Build mascara up more on the outer half of the eyelid.

Almond-set eyes

These are considered to be the perfect proportions and are well balanced in shape. This eye shape suits all make-up styles. Use eyeliner on the upper lid and make eyes appear big. Apply mascara to the upper lashes, emphasising the outer corners. Eyebrows should be well groomed to frame the eyes.

Large eyes
Be careful when applying eyeshadow, keep colour close to the lash line fading out towards the crease across the width of the eyelid. Do not shade in the crease or take colour above it. Matt colours suit large eyelids better.

Droopy eyelids
This can make the eyes look tired. Lighten under the outer corner of the eye with a highlighter. Line only the top lash line lifting the line slightly at the outer corner. Use a neutral shade over the lid and gradually get darker above the crease. Pay more attention to the outer half of the eye.

Hooded eyelids
The eyelid is mostly hidden by a fold of skin. Make sure you put eyeshadow on the eyelid as when you blink it will be visible if you have missed it. Soften the shadow towards the brow so there are no hard lines. Apply a lighter colour in the inner corner to open the eye.

LIPS

Full lips
Don't over line the lips.

Keep colour within the lip line.

Keep your colour soft for daytime; anything dark will bring attention to them.

Matt and gloss colours look best.

Thin lips
Shape the lips first. Using a line evens out the shape.

You can use rich colours within a line.

Use a small touch of shine in the middle.

Don't use dark colours.

Lip plumpers will increase the blood flow to the lips and make them appear fuller.

Small bowed lips
Use a liner to fill out the sides of the top lip slightly and to even out the shape.

Be careful using dark colours.

Accentuate the natural bow on the top lip. This is what everyone else wants!

Mature lips
Use a primer or cover your lips with a little foundation, and always use a liner. This stops the 'bleeding'.

Wide lips
Use a liner to emphasise the natural bow in the centre of the top lip. Matt lipsticks can make the lips look flat, so use a gloss to add depth.

Line outside the lip line if you want to play down the lips.

APPLYING FALSE TAN

The first thing you should think about when applying false tan is WHEN you should apply it. It's best to do it two nights before the event or job as then there is still plenty of time to cover up any mistakes. This also gives time for the chemical smell to disappear.

Now you need to prepare the skin – so even if you regularly body brush, it's still best to exfoliate around any dry areas of the body, paying particular attention to the knees, backs of heels, elbows and feet.

When coming out of the shower or bath, make sure you dry yourself really well, but also try to avoid getting too hot which could cause you to perspire and this could cause a streaky look.

Make sure you apply a good moisturiser all over the body, paying particular attention to the dry areas mentioned above. Allow the moisturiser to dry.

The bottle of false tan may have been sat on the shelf for a while, so shake well. If the ingredients have separated you could end up with an uneven tan!

Irrespective of which type of false tan you use – gel, spray or lotion – the best effect is achieved by using a circular motion as this will give the most even tan. Do not use in an up and down motion.

Don't forget to wash your hands regularly or you will get tanned palms. False tan has a tendency to sit in-between the fingers so don't forget to give them a scrub too.

Never apply false tan to the hands, feet elbows or knees. Use product from

---

JEANNE'S TOP TIPS

TRY NAIL MAGIC, AN EXCELLENT PRODUCT FOR DRY, BRITTLE AND SPLITTING NAILS. EVERY NIGHT FILE YOUR NAILS, JUST TAKING OFF ANY SMALL BREAKS. PAINT ON A LAYER OF NAIL MAGIC. ON THE 2ND DAY, PAINT ON A LAYER OF NAIL MAGIC. ON THE 3RD DAY, TAKE IT ALL OFF WITH NAIL POLISH REMOVER AND START FROM THE BEGINNING AGAIN. WHEN I DID THIS MY NAILS WERE BEAUTIFUL FOR MY WEDDING DAY, THE BEST THEY HAVE EVER BEEN.

a nearby area so you don't apply too much. When applying to the face and neck remember less is more and apply sparingly.

Once you have covered your whole body with false tan allow it all to dry for at least 15 minutes. Think about what to wear after your tan application. You don't want to ruin all that hard work. Wear loose-fitting clothes, preferably with no tight waistbands or cuffs, as these will rub off any false tan.

Products nowadays will come out of any clothes or linen on a normal 30 degree wash, but don't wear anything white!

BODY BRUSHING

This is a great way to stimulate your circulation and lymphatic systems and helps to eliminate toxins.

Body brushing not only improves the appearance of the skin, but also gives benefits to your health as it improves blood circulation and the immune systems.

You can get a body brush from most high street chemists costing as little as £3.00. Choose one with a long handle which will help to reach difficult areas such as the back. The brush has natural bristles and must always be kept dry.

The ideal time to brush is in the morning, before taking a shower. It is important to brush all areas except the face or any sensitive areas. It is vital to body brush in the right direction: always towards the heart. Use long smooth strokes on the arms, legs and buttocks, concentrating on the hips and thighs as this can also help to reduce the appearance of cellulite and dimpled skin.

Do it once every day then eventually it will become part of your beauty regime. When starting to body brush start with a small amount of pressure as the sensation takes a little getting used to, but it is invigorating. As you get used to it more pressure can be applied.

MAKE-UP BRUSHES

It is an idea to invest in a good, simple range of make-up brushes. There are many make-up brushes on the market. Here are a few examples, with the jobs that they do:

Foundation brush
This ensures an even application of foundation. Just a sweep of the brush on areas that need coverage. You could use a sponge to blend away any lines.

Concealer brush

This is usually slim and tapered for precision. You are able to apply a small amount of concealer onto the brush to cover up a small spot or blemish without affecting the foundation or base. You can use it also to cover dark circles under the eyes. An alternative to a concealer brush is YSL Touché Éclat. This is an excellent product and a must in every make-up bag. It covers up dark circles under the eyes and is like a pen (also known as the 'gold pen'). It sells for approximately £21 and can be bought from any good pharmacy or department store. Other companies sell their version, for example Art Deco.

> **TIFFANY'S TOP TIPS**
>
> ALWAYS TRY TO BUY FOUNDATION AND FACE MOISTURISING CREAM WITH A MINIMUM SPF 15, AND ALWAYS WEAR SUNCREAMS WITH A MINIMUM SPF 20 WHEN YOU ARE EXPOSED TO THE SUN.

Powder brush

This is used to apply loose powder over foundation. Typically, this is a brush medium to large in size with long bristles. These can also be used for blending in foundation and to eliminate make-up lines and cover blemishes.

Blusher brush

This brush is used to apply blusher to the cheeks. The bristles are long, soft and round in shape and allow easy application of blusher to large areas quickly and effortlessly. The brush is dabbed onto the blusher and then brushed over the apple of the cheeks, which gives an attractive hue and a burst of healthy colour to the face. Or you can apply to the under part of the cheekbones to bring out the visible line.

Shadow brush

This is the most common of brushes. The bristles are short and soft and it is used to apply eyeshadow to the main part of the eyelid. Sweep brush over eyeshadow and then stroke the brush over the eyelid.

Angled brush

This brush is used to apply the eyeshadow in to the crease of the eye. The angled brush bristles are short and soft and are angled for maximum usage. This brush is dabbed on to the eyeshadow and applied in to the crease of the lid. This brush is necessary to successfully achieve certain detailed looks, for example the 'Smokey eye look'.

Jeanne's Top Tips

FOR A STYLISH PORTFOLIO CASE, HAVE A PLAIN CASE WITH NO AGENCY LOGO ON. YOU CAN'T BE WITH MORE THAN ONE AGENCY IN ANY MAJOR CITY BUT IT DOESN'T LOOK GOOD ADVERTISING AN AGENCY FOR EXAMPLE IN BIRMINGHAM AT A CASTING FOR AN AGENCY IN LONDON. KEEP IT SIMPLE AND ELEGANT. WE SELL SOME GREAT ONES AT WWW.WANNABEWORKSHOPS.COM FOR A VERY COMPETITIVE PRICE.

Blending brush

This brush is used to blend in eyeshadow in order to promote a more natural, softer look. This brush is used to blend in where two shades of eyeshadow meet. It also removes excess shadow.

Eyebrow brush

This brush gives the eyebrows a fuller and more defined look. The bristles are firm and are medium to short in length. The eyebrow brush is dabbed over loose eyeshadow and applied gently and evenly over the eyebrows.

Lipstick brush

This is used to fill in the desired colour of the lips after the lip liner has been applied. This brush features short and firm bristles. The lipstick brush is used by gently dabbing the brush into desired lip colour and applying to lip.

Cleaning your brushes.

Make-up brushes can hold lots of dirt and bacteria but frequent washing can keep them, and your face, clean and healthy.

1. Run the brushes under warm water.

2. Apply a small amount of shampoo (for normal hair or baby) or an antibacterial wash, such as Carex.

3. Work into a light lather.

4. Rinse thoroughly under running water until the water runs clean.

5. Allow the brushes to air dry. Make sure your brushes dry flat – if they dry upright all the bristles will splay outwards. You can get specialised cleaning solutions to clean your brushes and these are available at most beauty supply stores.

If you find any stray hairs hanging out of your brush you can cut them off using a small, sharp pair of scissors. Be careful not to cut the rest of the bristles off!

Make-up brushes are sold by the make-up houses such as Clinique, Mac, Revlon, No7, No17, Christian Dior, Bobbi Brown, to name but a few. They are all found in reputable chemists, department stores, or look at www.crownbrush.co.uk where brushes can be bought online.

> **TIFFANY'S TOP TIPS**
>
> ALWAYS BE PUNCTUAL AND PROFESSIONAL AT ALL TIMES. YOU NEVER KNOW WHO IS WATCHING YOU.

EYEBROWS

Having your eyebrows plucked and groomed makes such a difference to your face, as these are what frame your eyes. You can have your eyebrows tweezed (using tweezers), waxed or the latest trend, threading, is a method which originated in Asia. Threading uses cotton to remove the hairs.

Well-groomed eyebrows are key to a striking look; however, the biggest mistake people make is to tweeze them too much. Avoid over plucking as it takes a long time for the hairs to grow back.

The space between your eyebrows should be a little wider than your eyes or equal to it. Take a long eyeshadow brush or pencil and hold it parallel to the side of your nose, where the brush meets your brow is where your eyebrow should begin.

Extend the brush diagonally from your nostril, following the outside edge of your eye towards the brow. Where the inside of the brush hits is where your brows should end.

The best eyebrows have a small arch. To find yours, hold the brush or pencil parallel to the outside edge of the coloured part of the eye (iris). Where the brush meets the brow is where the highest part of your eyebrow should be.

If you are going to tweeze, and to do it yourself invest in a good pair of tweezers with a slanted edge. Make sure you are near a good natural light and it's best to use a magnifying mirror. Keep checking the overall look in a normal mirror.

Hold skin taut and pluck hairs in the direction that they grow, this will be less painful. Ensure that you pluck each hair individually. Take your time for best results.

Some people say never tweeze from the top but this is a myth. However, just be careful not to over pluck from this area.

For men

Sometimes with men's eyebrow shaping, all that is needed is to trim. This helps keep the hairs in place and makes the look lighter and well groomed. Often men end up taking away hair that does not need to be. To keep eyebrows in check, trim every 3-4 weeks.

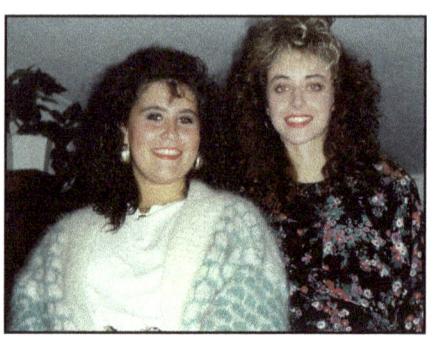

Friends Tiffany and Zoe Tyler, a TV celebrity and voice coach.

We recommend that you visit a beauty therapist to have your eyebrows professionally shaped for the first time. An eyebrow shape in a salon costs around £9. Once you have the initial shape it will be easy for you to maintain it yourself. If you want to reduce the discomfort, a good tip is to take a couple of painkillers like Neurofen about 20 minutes before the treatment. It is also very important to ensure the skin around your eyes is clean and clear of make-up before and after removing hair, otherwise clogged pores, ingrown hairs and painful spots may occur. It is common for the brow area to redden. A cooling gel like aloe vera will help to reduce this; however this usually clears on its own after an hour or two. Due to redness it is a good idea to shape eyebrows the day before a casting or job.

HOW TO LOOK AFTER YOUR NAILS

Strong nails make for stunning hands. Here are a few simple steps to help you achieve this.

1. Get rid of all traces of nail polish using an acetone-free remover.

2. Rinse each hand immediately so that the remover does not stay in contact with your nails too long as this tends to dry them out.

3. Soak your hands in warm soapy water for a few minutes.

4. Remove the dead skin from around the nails.

5. Once the hands are dry, bathe them in olive oil to nourish and strengthen the nail's keratin (basic substance of your nail).

6. Next run a nail buffer over your nails to remove ridges and give your nails a natural looking shine.

7. To file the nail start from the outside and work in towards the centre. Always go in the same direction to help avoid splitting. Never use a metal nail file as this weakens the nail.

NAILS

8. Apply a moisturiser, massaging it into the hands and nails.

9. If you are applying a coloured nail varnish always use a base coat first: this helps to prevent staining.

Strengthening

If your nails are brittle or flaky, avoid growing them too long. Cut them square and quite short. Massage them every night with special nail creams, or with a bit of olive oil, to prevent them from splitting.

> **JEANNE'S TOP TIPS**
>
> MOISTURISE YOUR BODY – APPLY A BODY LOTION ALL OVER THE BODY AFTER EVERY SHOWER OR BATH, PAYING PARTICULAR ATTENTION TO THE ELBOWS, KNEES AND THE BACKS OF YOUR HEELS. THIS KEEPS THE SKIN SUPPLE AND REDUCES THE SIGNS OF AGEING AND STRETCH MARKS.

Maintaining

You need to look after your cuticles regularly to keep your nails healthy. These are the little bits of skin that protect the base of the nail getting torn easily. After you have massaged your nails with cream, gently push back the cuticle using an orange stick or cotton wool bud.

Protecting

In order to protect your nails, use products that are specifically designed to treat them. Care for brittle nails with fortifying, hardening care products. Look after nails that have broken with strengthening care products. Use nourishing varnish on dry nails.

Choosing a varnish

This final step, choosing the varnish, is personal choice. The varnish can be purely aesthetic but it can also help solve such problems as hardness or splitting. There are varnishes available that harden the keratin and prevent the nails from breaking.

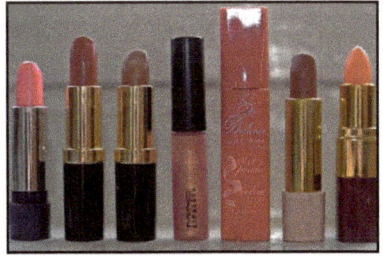

1. Don't bite your nails! There are special nail varnishes to help as they have a bitter taste.

2. Avoid cutting your nails, file them.

3. Try not to use varnishes that are quick dry as these weaken the nail.

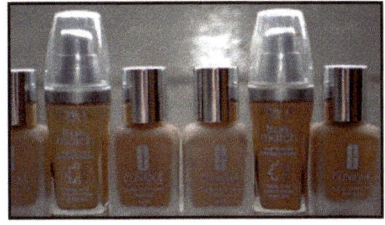

4. Always use a protective base coat underneath coloured varnish.
5. Always wear gloves for washing up, gardening etc.
6. Use a hand cream which also protects the nails.

If you are about to go on a modelling job never use any nail varnishes other than a nude, natural colour or a clear. Using a strong colour will automatically date a photograph. It may also clash with the clothes you have been given to model!

Nowadays you don't have to make do with the nails that you have. There are so many different fashionable options available.

Here we outline some of the available choices:

Acrylic nails

Also known as false, fake and extensions. This is a covering that is placed over the natural nail to enhance it. There are two different options with acrylic nails: tips or forms.

Tips are lightweight plastic plates that are nail shaped. They are glued on to the end of your natural nail and an acrylic is then applied to the whole nail covering the tip. The nail is then painted as in a normal manicure. The acrylic nail will last approximately four weeks, but the polish may need to be re-applied.

A form is made up of a mixture of polymer powder and a liquid monomer which starts to harden 30-40 seconds after application and continues to harden for a further 15 minutes. Another material is also used called a UV top coat, where the polymer resin hardens under a UV light. These are more flexible, last longer but are more expensive.

As with all substitute nails, an acetone-free nail polish remover needs to be used when just taking off the polish. After approximately four weeks you have the option to have infills or have the acrylic soaked off. A full set of acrylic nails costs approximately £40, with infills costing about £30.

Approximately after every five infills you decide whether you want to take them off and give your natural nails the time to breathe or start from scratch again. With acrylic nails you need special products to soak off and at no point should they be picked off. This causes damage and distress to the natural nail.

There is also the option of wraps. This is where a silk or fibreglass overlay is placed over the natural nail. This is more commonly used if the client is allergic to any of the chemicals found in the acrylic or gel nails. As the name suggests the nail is wrapped with the silk or fibre glass and then covered with a resin or glue. If you have a good length nail, but suffer with brittle or splitting nails, this is a good option. Starting price for wraps is about £30.

Gel Nails

These were designed as an alternative to nail extensions and are less distressing to the natural nail. Here, several layers of a gel polish are put on the nail and after each layer they are set under a UV light which hardens and sets

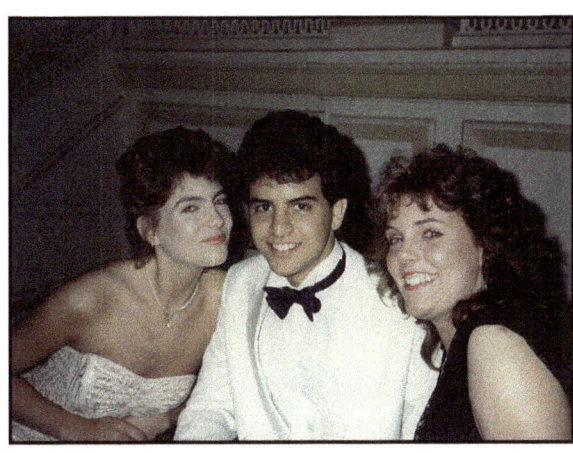

Jeanne in the Miss UK competition with Glen Maderos and her sister.

the gel. This protects your own nail, and allows it time to grow. Colours are limited, but this process is getting more and more popular. The gel nails last approximately 10-14 days and cost from £25 a set. Companies that do gel nails are www.biosculpt.co.uk, www.Jessica-Nails.co.uk and www.shellacnailscnd.com. You can paint over gel nails with a coloured polish, but again you must use an acetone-free polish. When the gel nails need to come off never pick them off; they need to be soaked off properly to avoid damaging the natural nail. You can buy your own home kit to put gel on your own nails and this costs approximately £54.

Nail Art

Nail art are designs that are painted onto your nail. The beautician will use a variety of colours and different nibbed pens to achieve swirls, patterns and even animals or birds. Crystals can be used also; they are attached by special nail glue.

Minx

This is a company that uses a transfer straight on the nail. Again, similar to the silk and fibreglass wrap, the transfer is placed over the nail and then cut to fit. This is fairly difficult to do as you must get the transfer lying flat on the nail. Heat is used to set the minx. A set of minx nails costs approximately £35 and to find a stockist near you check out www.minxnails.com. The transfer designs can be very beautiful, from a liquid gold or silver to tiger prints and spots.

HEALTHY DIET

The following are the basic guidelines for a nutritious, healthy diet.

1. Eat plenty of high fibre foods such as fruits, vegetables, beans and wholegrain. These are good carbohydrates. They are nutritious, filling and relatively low in calories. They should supply the 20-30 grams of dietary fibre you need each day, which slows the absorption of carbohydrates, so there's less of a detrimental effect on insulin and blood sugar levels. It also provides other health benefits too. Such foods provide important vitamins, minerals and plant chemicals essential for healthy skin, hair and bones.

2. Make sure you include the foods naturally coloured green, orange and yellow into your diet. Foods like broccoli, carrots and citrus fruits. The antioxidants and other nutrients in these foods may help protect against developing certain cancers and diseases. Eat five or more portions of fruit or vegetables a day.

3. Limit the intake of sugary foods – refined sugars such as white bread and salty snacks. Sugar is our number one additive – it is added to a wide variety of foods, some of which you would be shocked about. Many sugary foods are also high in fat, so are calcium dense.

4. Cut down on animal fats. These foods are rich in saturated fats which boost cholesterol levels and can cause other health problems. Choose lean meats, skinless chicken and non-fat or low fat dairy products.

5. Cut down on trans fat which is found in hydrogenated vegetable oils, used in most processed foods and many fast foods. Check food labels!

6. Eat more fish and nuts, which contain certain healthy unsaturated fats. Use olive oil instead of butters and margarines.

7. Keep portions moderate. Over the years our portion sizes have got considerably larger.

8. Keep your cholesterol intake around 300 milligrams per day. Cholesterol is found only in animal products i.e. meat, poultry, dairy products and egg yolks.

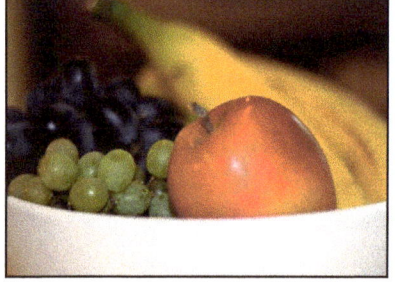

9. Eat a variety of foods. Don't eat the same things every day. It is possible that not every essential nutrient has been identified, so eating a wide range of foods ensures that you are getting all the necessary nutrients.

This will also limit your exposure to pesticides and toxic substances that could be found in one particular food.

10. Maintain an adequate intake of calcium. Calcium is essential for healthy bones and teeth. It is found in all low fat sources such as skimmed milk and low fat yoghurts. If you feel you are not getting the right amount you could always take a supplement.

11. Having said the above, try to get your vitamins and minerals from a healthy diet and *not* from supplements. A healthy diet also supplies nutrients and other compounds as well as vitamins and minerals. Food also provides the 'synergy' that nutrients require to be efficiently used in the body.

12. Maintain a healthy weight. Try and balance calorie intake with energy output. Exercise and physical activity is essential.

13. If you drink alcohol, do it in moderation. That is one drink a day for women, and two for men. A drink = 12 ounces of beer, 4 ounces of wine, 1.5 ounces of an 80% proof spirit. Drinking in excess causes many health issues and adds additional calories to your diet without supplying any nutrients.

14. Drink plenty of water, at least eight glasses a day. Plenty of water helps keep your skin, body and muscles hydrated.

This does not mean you have to give up your favourite foods. As long as you're overall diet is balanced and rich in nutrients and fibre there is nothing wrong with the odd cheeseburger. Just limit how often you have one and try to eat moderate amounts of your 'treats'.

EXERCISE

There are 1,440 minutes in a day and you only need to exercise for 30 minutes of them a day.

Exercise is so important in staying healthy. People who are active generally live longer and feel better. Exercise can help you maintain a healthy weight. It can delay or prevent health problems such as diabetes 2, some cancers and heart disease. Most adults need 30 minutes of physical activity a day at least five days a week. You could do a brisk walk, mow the lawn, dance, swim or cycle. Stretching and weight training can also strengthen the body and improve your fitness level.

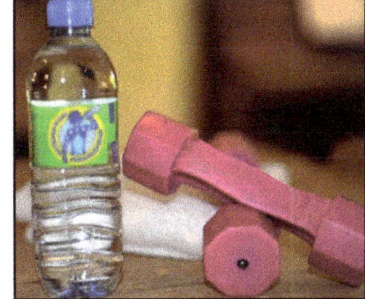

Tiffany's Top Tips

TRY AND MAKE SURE YOU DRINK PLENTY OF WATER A DAY (8 GLASSES) AND GET AT LEAST 8 HOURS SLEEP PER NIGHT.

The key to exercise is to find an activity that best suits you and your lifestyle. If you enjoy whatever you decide to do you are likely to stick with it. You could ask a friend; go running together or join a class, and you will motivate each other.

There are so many different types of exercises available to you. It doesn't mean you have to pound the streets or a gym. There are so many classes that are taking the country by storm.

Here are a few available and a brief description:

Zumba – this is a Latin dance-inspired fitness programme created by Alberto 'Beto' Perez from Columbia. It involves dance and aerobic elements and the choreographer incorporates Hip Hop, Soca, Samba, Salsa, Merengue, Mambo, as well as Martial Arts. It also uses Bollywood moves and belly dancing and incorporates lunges and squats for an all round workout.

Body attack – this is a cardio workout that builds up your stamina and strength. It is a high energy interval training programme that combines athletic aerobic movements with strength, as well as using stabilisation exercises. Body Attack is aimed at the weekend athlete and the hard core competitor. Dynamic instructors and powerful music empower you to achieve your goal.

Body balance – this is an exercise that lasts for an hour. It is a programme where beautiful music is used to do a range of stretches, poses and balances. It is part tai chi, yoga and pilates. It builds up strength and flexibility and leaves you feeling centred and calm.

Body combat – this is a workout where you are totally unleashed. It is a fierce programme using a wide range of moves from tae kwon do, tai chi, karate and boxing. Powerful music and dynamic instructors take you through combat.

Body pump – this is a class where the barbell is used. In 60 minutes you use all the major muscle groups doing exercises such as squats, press lifts and curls. All done to music, your choice of weight inspires you to get the results you require, and fast.

Yoga and pilates – these are holistic classes that help improve your suppleness and flexibility. They are an excellent choice to relieve stress and keep fit at the same time.

Strength and conditioning classes – these are perfect for toning up your muscles and sculpting your body the way you want it to be.

Step classes – an aerobic-based workout using an elevated platform. The height of the step can be chosen by you. Many gyms and fitness centres offer a step class. It normally lasts 60 minutes.

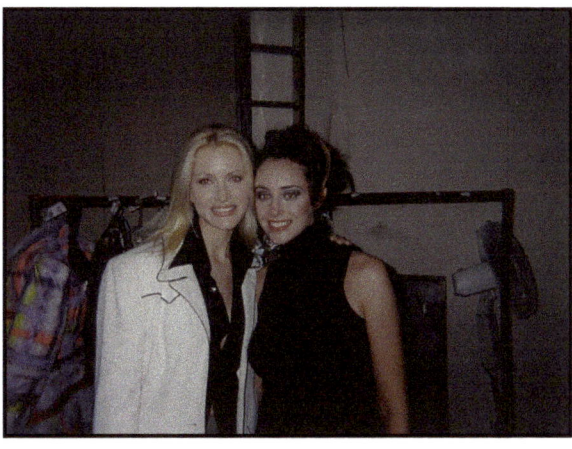

Tiffany with Caprice, late 90s.

Circuit training – this is normally a course that covers upper body exercise such as press-ups, bench dips, pull-ups, core exercises (e.g. sit-ups, stomach crunches) and lower body exercises (e.g. squat jumps, step-ups, compass jumps). When one circuit is complete, you begin the circuit again.

Gymphobics – a ladies only gym. Here a 30 minute-exercise programme is done on different pieces of equipment. You are allocated a time for each machine and a timer goes when it is time to move to the next machine. It costs approximately £30 per month and recommended use is three times a week. It's great if you need to lose a substantial amount of weight or if you feel self-conscious and just want to be with other females. Check out www.gymphobics.co.uk for your local gyms and a free guest pass.

Everyone is different and what makes you happy and suits you and your body doesn't necessary suit everyone. Running is a good all-rounder for the body, as is swimming. Try different classes and find a class that suits you. If you don't have the money to go to a class (approximately £4 per class) or to be a member of a gym (memberships range from £25-£80 depending on what gym and the times you want to go – note the busiest times for gyms are after work from 5.30-8pm which is classed as peak time) there are some great DVDs that are endorsed by celebrities. Davina McCall has an excellent exercise DVD. It has three 30-minute routines that work all the major muscle groups. Cindy Crawford's first video is brilliant. Although it's a slightly longer programme at 40 minutes, there is no travel time to add on to your workout! DVDs cost approximately £12 and you will need to exercise at least three times a week and have a healthy diet too.

USEFUL CONTACTS

We have not listed any contact numbers due to constant changes in circumstances in model agencies, child agencies, promotional agencies, photographers who test, make-up artists and helpful websites' details. Please come to one of our Wannabe Workshops where you can receive all the recent correct business details of reputable and legitimate companies that we have worked with or know:

www.wannabeworkshops.com

BEAUTY COMPETITIONS

During our modelling careers we have entered various beauty competitions and, between us, won a few.

In fact Tiffany got into the modelling industry by entering her first beauty competition 'Miss West Midlands' in 1988 (Jeanne was in it too!) and by making friends with the other competitors Tiffany got advice and model agency numbers.

Beauty competitions aren't as popular now as they were in our hay day, due to political correctness, but they are slowly making a comeback and fortunately all the big UK competitions still exist. Here are some useful names and websites of various beauty competitions currently running:

www.missgreatbritain.co.uk – various heats are held all around the UK in different regions, e.g. Worcester, Kent, Wolverhampton, Liverpool. You can enter the heats by filling in the registration forms online. The winner of Miss Great Britain will go onto represent her country in the American beauty pageant 'Miss Universe'. CEO Kate Solomon.

www.missengland.info – again, this is entered through heats in different regions around England and the winner will represent her country in 'The Miss World' pageant.

www.teenqueenuk.com – you can enter this competition online.

www.universegb.co.uk

www.missteengreatbritain.co.uk

www.mistersuperinternational.com

www.missspiritoftruebeauty.com

www.missindiaworldwide.uk

BEAUTY COMPETITIONS

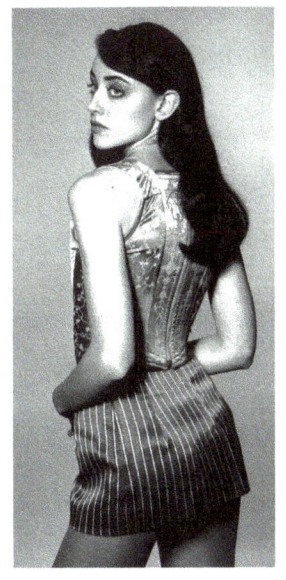

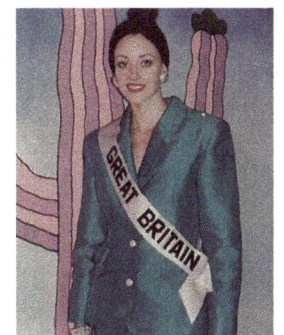

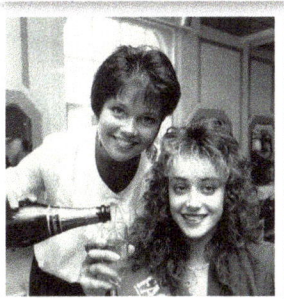

*Top left: Tiffany's publicity shot used for the 'New Miss British Isles' competition, taken by John Stoddard and clothes by Vivienne Westwood. She leant me a massive wardrobe to take to the Miss Universe pageant in Thailand for a month.
Top right: Tiffany as Miss Great Britain in Thailand.
Middle right: Winning Face of the Midlands in 1988.*

*Right: Winning Miss Beautiful Eyes in 1991 at London Zoo. Who did actually win, can you guess?
Bottom right: Tiffany and roommate Miss Guam in Thailand.
Below As Face of the Midlands on a billboard in Birmingham for one year.*

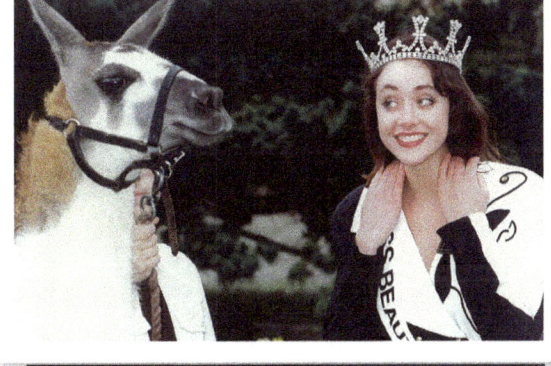

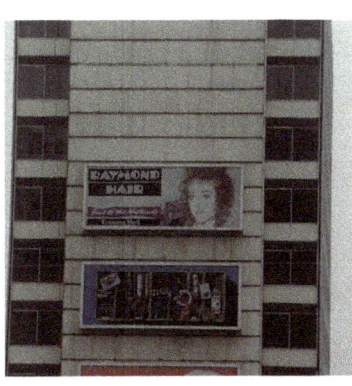

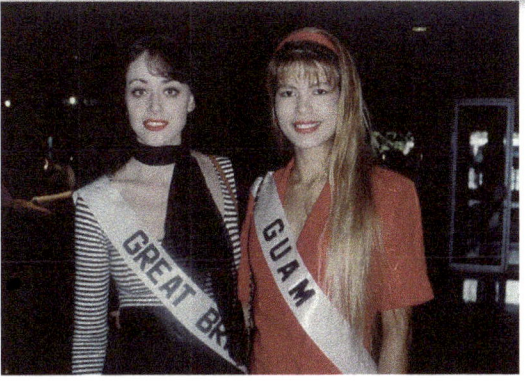

www.galaxypageantsuk.com
www.missearthgirls.co.uk
www.misslimo.com

Because beauty competitions change all the time, it can be useful to do a bit of 'Google searching' for current competitions.

We sponsor Miss Great Britain and Miss Spirit of True Beauty and take part as judges.

Tiffany didn't win every competition she entered, but was usually placed. She won:

'Face of the Midlands' 1988.

'Miss Beautiful Eyes' 1991

'Miss British Isles' 1992, after which she went on to represent her country as 'Miss Great Britain' in the American pageant 'Miss Universe' in Thailand, 1992.

As a 'Miss Great Britain' winner, Tiffany went on to be a guest judge at some beauty competitions, at 'Miss Hawaiian tropic' in Nottingham, and 'Miss Great Britain' 1998, where she sat next to Simon Cowell, who was also on the judging panel! She was also guest judge at the 'Miss Wolverhampton' heat for Miss Great Britain in 2010.

Jeanne didn't win every competition she entered but was usually placed, she won:

'Miss Kidderminster' 1986

'Miss Photographic' 1989

'Miss Quarybank' 1989. (In 1990 Jeanne was a guest judge on the judging panel.)

'Miss BRMB' 1989

'Miss Birmingham' 1989

'Miss Superstore' 1989

'Miss Merry Hill' 1991

You can win some amazing prizes. Between us, we have won holidays, clothes, money, jewellery, make-up, vouchers and luggage.

There are also some special model agency competitions that you might find in magazines, so keep a lookout for these and also for TV competitions e.g. 'Britain's next top Model'.

Some potential models can get lucky and are scouted by people from agencies around the UK and at places like 'The Clothes Show' in Birmingham, which is a popular place to go and to get spotted!

Beauty Competitions

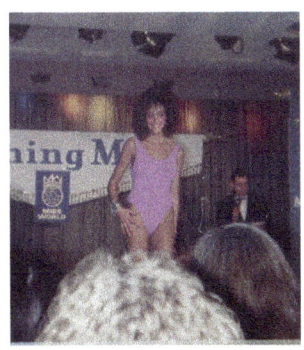

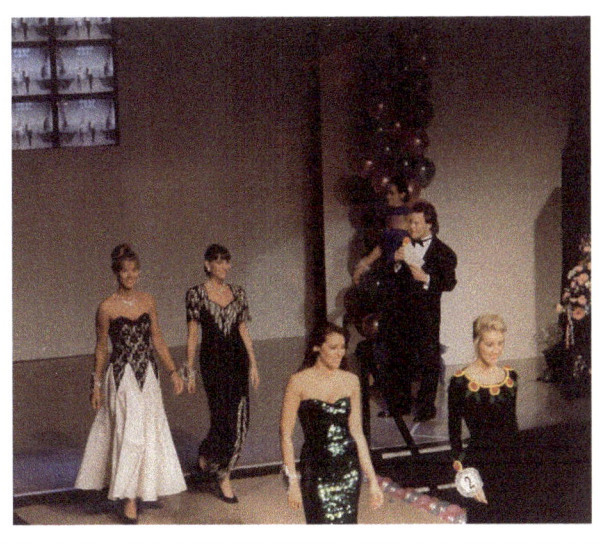

Top left: Tiffany in Miss West Midlands 1988.
Top right: Jeanne in Miss UK final. Bruno Brookes as compère.
Right: Jeanne's first beauty competition. Winning Miss Kidderminster.
Below: Tiffany on brochure for Miss Universe 1992.
Bottom right: Tiffany in Thailand for Miss Universe, looking like a giant next to the local girls.

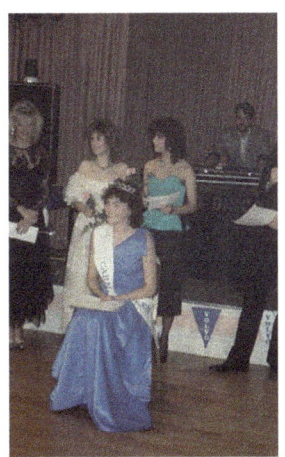

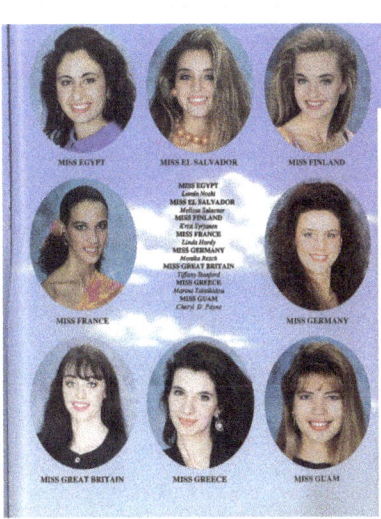

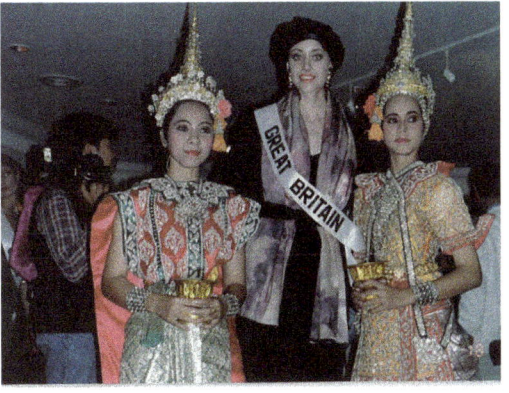

EXAMPLE INVOICE

ADDRESS:
    Wannabe Workshops,
    PO Box 6059,
    Kidderminster,
    31.05.10

INVOICE TO:
    Richard Smith,
    Walkers lane,
    Solihull,
    West midlands,
    B73 2AT.

NUMBER: 04762

JOB: 31stMay 2010 Half day photo shoot

TOTAL DUE: £130.00

PAYMENT: All cheques to be payable to Miss J Frith and sent to the address above. Thank you for this booking.

GLOSSARY

Accessories – *jewellery, tights, belts, bags, hats etc.*

Admin charges – *charges made to you by an agency to cover paperwork that it will have done for you. This also includes stamps and envelopes to send out cheques for jobs.*

Buyout fee – *an extra fee paid on top of your day rates so the client can use the shots for extra promotional material, or for a certain length of time e.g. six months or a year.*

Castings – *a time and place booked by a client to see potential models who could be suitable for an available job. They basically want to meet you in the* *flesh (an audition). A requested casting is even better to go to as they have specifically asked to see you.*

Commercial photography – *photography that will end up on billboards, buses and posters etc. Photography to sell a product e.g. sofas or a computer.*

Composite card – *normally an A5 card with a head and shoulder shot on the front and on the back lots of different shots including work pictures, body shots and any specialised parts e.g. legs. All your details, including height and measurements, will be on here.*

Direct work – *work that you do without being represented by an agency.*

Disc – *this is a computer disc that you may get your test shots on.*

Editorial photography – *where your shots will be used in magazines or even the cover.*

Fashion photography – *where the job is all about the clothes.*

Fittings – *a job where you try on clothes so the client can see the general fit of the clothes.*

Glamour modelling – *topless or nude work.*

Go-sees – *a visit to a photographer's studio or an advertising agency to show them your portfolio in case a job comes in that you may be suitable for in the foreseeable future.*

Location – *when you will be working outside of a studio.*

Mini book – *mini version of your portfolio that is always kept at the agency, so that they can show it to their clients.*

Model release form – *a form that you will need to sign to release all rights to the pictures over to the client.*

Mother agent – *your main agency (usually in London) who will represent you; other agencies woud have to go through the Mother agency to give you any work.*

Portfolio – *a display case or book to show all your prints, from test shoots, tear sheets and any work shots that you have managed to get.*

Provisional – *a possible job. This is not a definite booking.*

Tear sheets – *your work shots, which you have torn out of a magazine, catalogue or newspaper to use in your portfolio.*

Tests – *a photographic session with a photographer, which you either pay for or get done for free. At the end you should get shots for your portfolio.*

Website – *the agency will have its own website and they will put your pictures on it for a fee.*

JEANNE'S FUNNY MODELLING STORIES

I only ever called in sick on a job once and that was when I had another job to go to on the same day! Once I had done it I was so worried that I would get caught that all the way to the train station in the taxi I laid down on the floor! When I got to my job, which was a Janet Raeger underwear show, and once we had all done our fitting, they suddenly announced: "We have all the papers here wanting to do a press call, so will you all please put on your first outfit and go outside!" It wasn't just any paper – there was *The Sun*, *Daily Mail*, and *The Independent*. So we all went outside and there were about 15 girls so I got right at the back and tried to hide. Suddenly one photographer pipes up: "Excuse me, you at the back, can we do some single shots of you please?" Just because my outfit was white with little red hearts all over it and it was Valentine's day that week! It was just typical, but luckily it didn't go in the paper until a few days later, so I got away with it. But, trust me, I never ever called in sick again. The stress was not worth any amount of money!!

When you put your specialities on a composite card it is BEST to always tell the truth. I was booked for a 50s look photo shoot. They wanted me to be on roller skates. I did make it VERY clear to my agent that I could NOT roller skate, but I did have some skates that I could borrow. When we got to the carpark where we were shooting it was a club in Dudley and it was covered in broken glass. The client said that they wanted the 50s car to be driving around with me holding on to the car door. Obviously, I laughed to start with, thinking they were joking, but apparently not! Anyway, they soon got the picture when I came out of the changing rooms walking like a crab, very slowly towards them. I am sure the agency on that occasion bent the truth a little!

When you are a model, nothing is private. A friend was on an underwear shoot when the client shouts out: "Hold on, she's just got a thread that I need to cut off." So she runs on set, grabs the thread, pulls it to cut…Well it was her tampax string! There were a few red faces.

When I was testing with a photographer we did some shots with my legs in the air and me on my shoulder blades. This shot was great and got me so much work. But even the photographer doesn't know this as luckily he had his stereo up really loud. Every time I pulled my legs down I did a huge fanny fart, which was totally out of my control. Well, I got a big hosiery contract and on a shoot they said they wanted to try and recreate the shot in my portfolio. There were at least 10 people – several clients, the photographer, plus his assistant, the make-up artist, stylist…the list was endless, but NO loud

Funny Stories

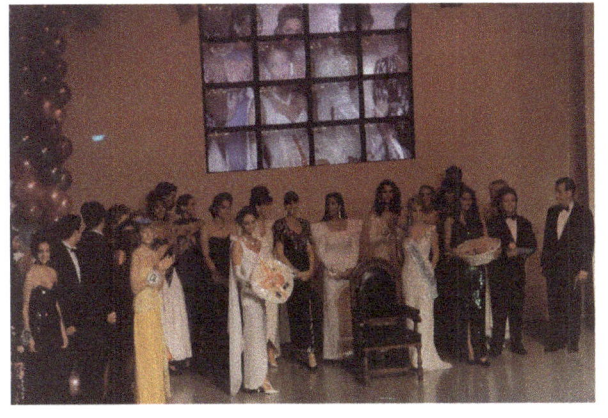

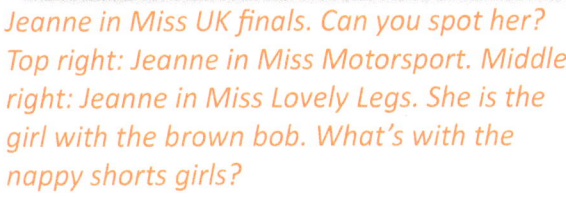

Jeanne in Miss UK finals. Can you spot her? Top right: Jeanne in Miss Motorsport. Middle right: Jeanne in Miss Lovely Legs. She is the girl with the brown bob. What's with the nappy shorts girls?
Below: Jeanne Miss Quarry Bank.
Bottom left: Jeanne doing charity fun run. Bottom right: Jeanne judging a competition.

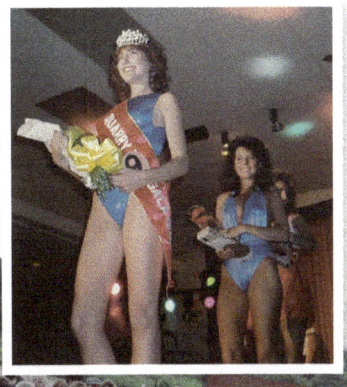

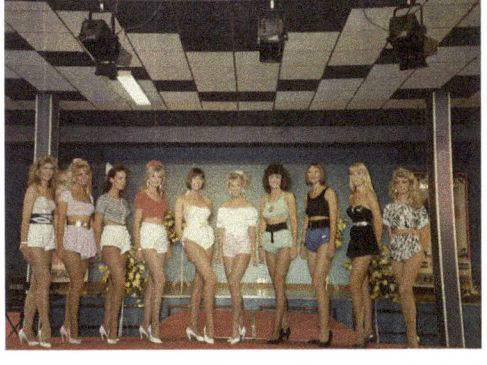

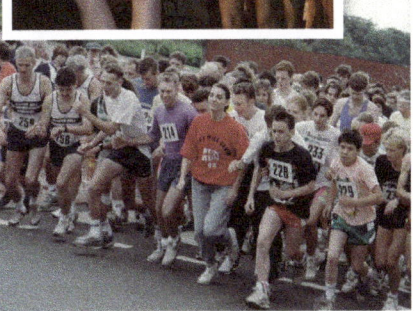

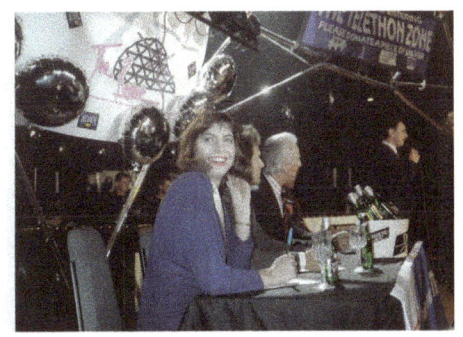

music. In fact, it was so quiet you could hear a pin drop, so I started to have a panic attack. I thought the best thing was to explain…For a while, no one said anything and you could see them trying to work out if what I had said was what they thought I had said. What made it worse was that I needn't have have been that honest, as I never fanny farted once on that shoot!!

I am never a diva, there is no point, but one day I was at a casting in London. As always with castings I had felt obliged to go. It costs so much money in trains, petrol, parking, underground and so on, so I had a got a cheap day return. Well, the clients kept me waiting for at least an hour and I had thought I would have been in and out. So I started to get a bit shirty. I said if they didn't see me, I would have to go. They were lovely and said they were sorry and would see me straightaway. I followed them to an office which was down some stairs in a basement office. I fell from the top of the stairs right down to the bottom, ending up upside down in a heap. I got up quickly and went and sat down at the desk. The first thing they said was: "Well we need someone who can walk well!" When I got on the train my knee was so swollen and I was so disappointed, having made such an effort and blown it. Two days later I got a call to say I'd got the job! I am now always tempted to collapse on every casting now, as it least it makes you stand out from the crowd!!

TIFFANY'S FUNNY MODELLING STORIES

During all the many fun and fabulous years of my modelling career I have many, many funny stories I could share with you, but there really are too many to mention them all. Apart from the usual tripping on the catwalk usually wearing far too long dresses, these are two of my favourite ones that made me laugh a lot!

I was doing a regular fashion show held in Birmingham and was modelling some fairly funky clothing and one of the outfits I had to wear was a pair of leatherette chaps with a tight bodysuit underneath. Now, in most fashion showcases, we models have very little room backstage and very little time to get changed, and this show was no exception. I was ready to go onto the stage, which I did in my usual professional manner and, whilst strutting, I could hear a few gasps and titters from some members of the audience. I didn't think anything of it and carried on walking, but when I was backstage one of the models said: "Tiff, part of your vagina and all of your pubes are hanging out at the side of the bodysuit" Mmm lovely. It was only then that I realised what the titters had been for!!

BEAUTY COMPETITIONS

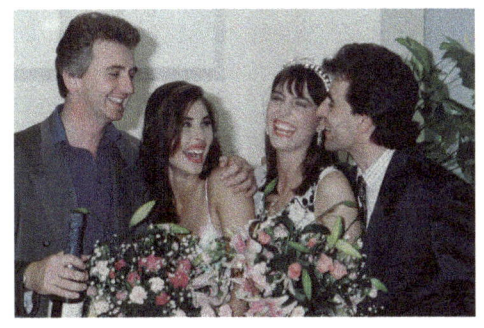

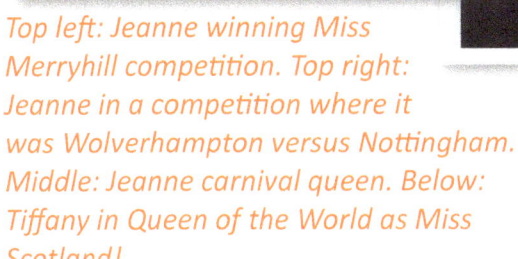

Top left: Jeanne winning Miss Merryhill competition. Top right: Jeanne in a competition where it was Wolverhampton versus Nottingham. Middle: Jeanne carnival queen. Below: Tiffany in Queen of the World as Miss Scotland!
Bottom: Tiffany left front row in a German magazine whilst competing in Queen of the World beauty competition 95.

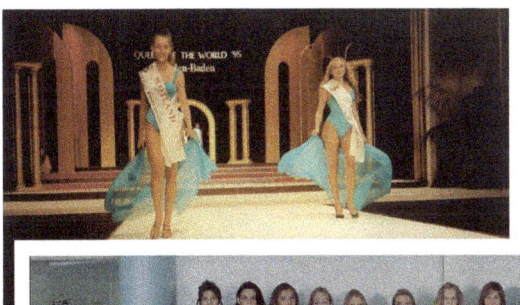

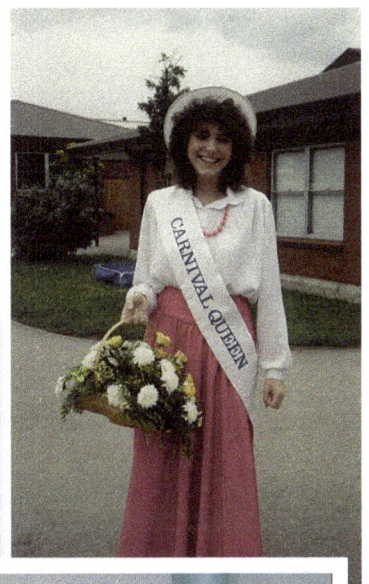

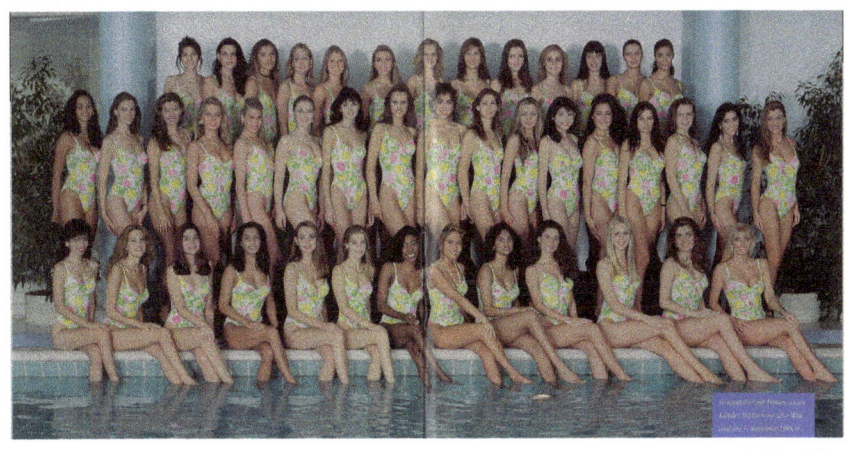

Do You Wannabe a Model? 114

The other story that I still laugh about is when I was doing stand modelling at the NEC in Birmingham at Premier Collections for some new young designers. The shows meant a lot to the young designers, who were so very excited when a buyer from a very big well-known UK department store took interest in the collection and wanted to know more about it. I had modelled all the collection and the designer was going through the available colour ranges when I heard him say: "'And this dress is also available in sage and onion?" Bless him. He had meant to say sage! I had to move away quickly as I just lost it with my laughter. How the buyer from the department store kept a straight face I do NOT know!!

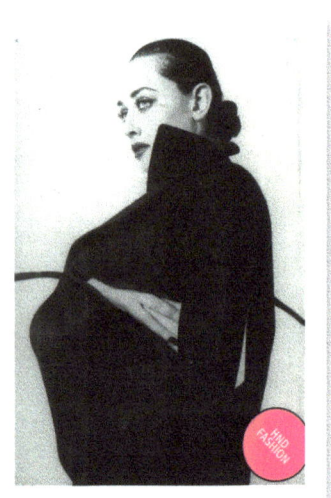
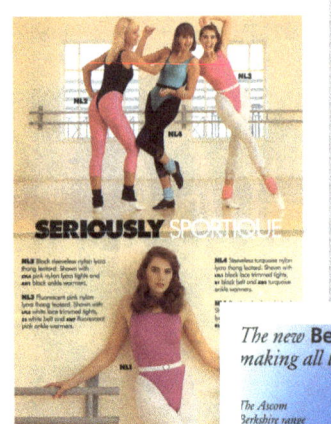
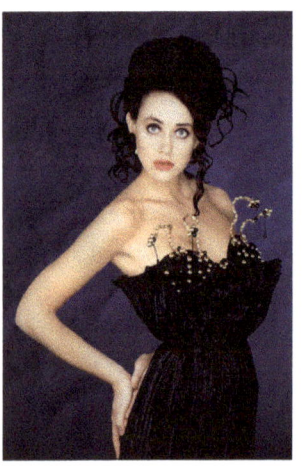

Clockwise from top left: Tiffany modelling a fashion student's design. What's with the claw finger!? Jeanne having fun modelling sportswear- Kids from Fame style! Jeanne modelling for Ascom Telecom. Tiffany modelling for different hair magazines...it is her own hair!

Jeanne's and Tiffany's Modelling Work

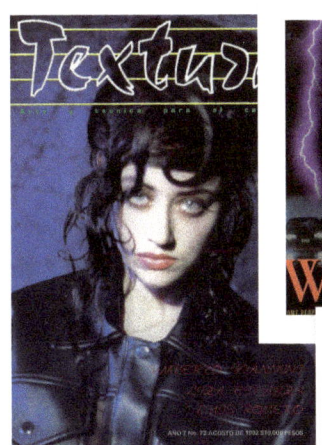
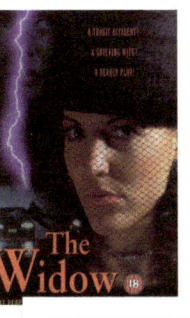
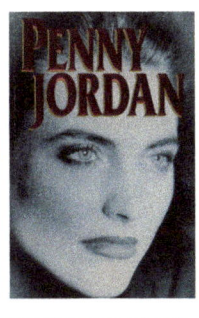
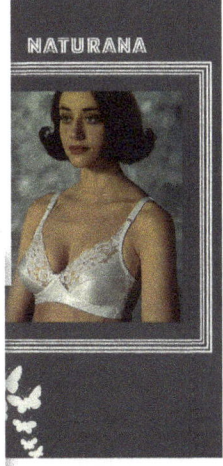
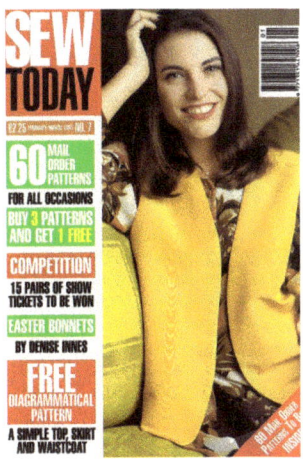
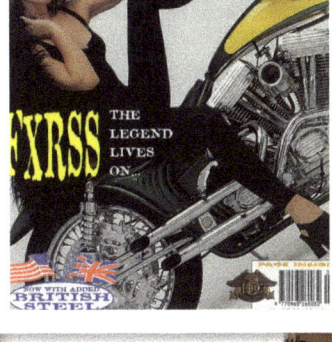
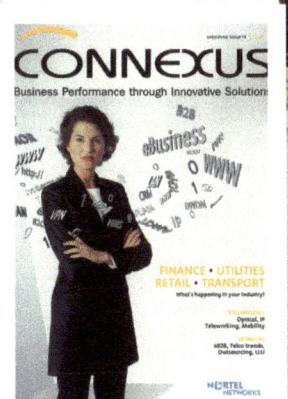
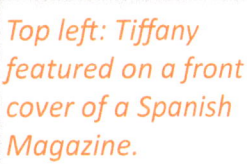
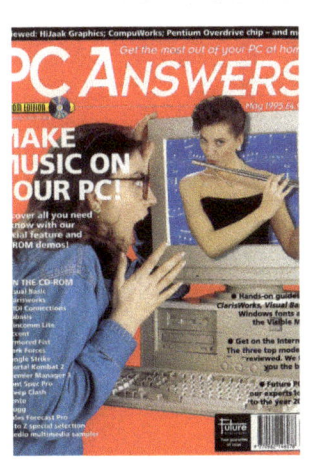

Top left: Tiffany featured on a front cover of a Spanish Magazine.
Top middle: Jeanne on a DVD cover and book cover shot. Top right: Bra packaging job by Tiffany for Naturana. Check the hair out. Left and middle: Jeanne's favourite cover shots. Top of the list involves a bike. Mellow Yellow – a fun modelling job for Tiffany.

DO YOU WANNABE A MODEL?

JEANNE'S MODELLING DIARY

Here is an extract from my Diary the year 2000 A week of work.

November 5th

This is the last day of a 5 day fashion show at the N.E.C Birmingham. We are doing regular shows throughout a golf exhibition. It's a choreographed show and there are about 10 models on the job. We are working roughly 9.30-6.00. The show lasts approximately 30 mins. It's good fun and the catwalk is like a golf course, it has astro turf on it and is a square shape and is not the traditionally catwalk. We are at floor level so people can get a good look at our golfing outfits as they walk past the show.

Monday 6th

I am on a full day Bridal shoot for Sallie Bee. I have booked all the other models for Sallie and sorted out a make up artist. I have worked for Sallie since I was 16 and I am now 30. She is a great client, strict but fair. It will be

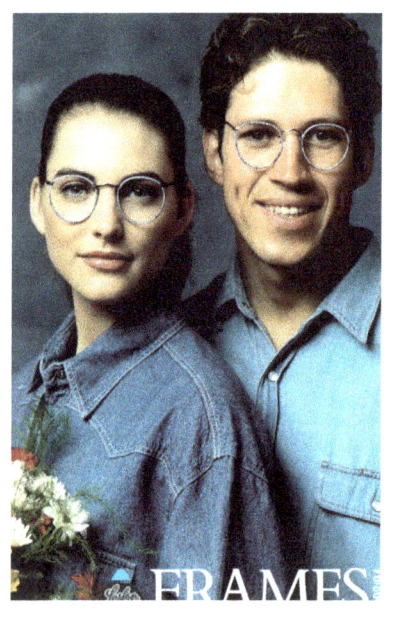

Jeanne modelling for a glasses company.

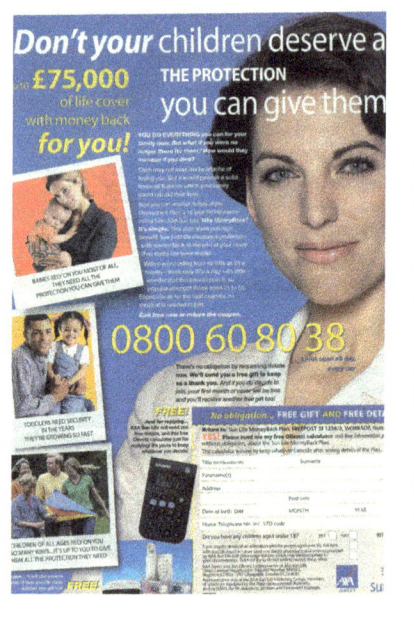

Jeanne commercial modelling for Sunlife – loving the short hair!

a long day 9.00 - 7 ish and the studio gets very cold. I have suffered with very bad chill blains and last time I worked I had to go straight to bed as I couldn't walk, its the very flimsy bridal shoes on such a cold concrete floor. I get to wear wedding dresses all day. It is a hard job as once you get into a position the photographer doesn't like me to move very much as Sallie likes the dress without any creases.

Tuesday 7th

I am in Surrey today for a job for BMA. I have to be there for 9am so I have left around 5am. I am to do my own hair and make up and take some shoes. I will be wearing uniforms.

Wednesday 9th

I have most of the day off, so I have been to the gym for a few hours and walked my dog, time to wash some clothes and pack away some of my shoes. I have to leave at 5.30 as I have a show tonight in Cardiff. It's a straight show with a choreographed beginning and end. I have to do my own make up and hair and take some shoes. I get home at 1am.

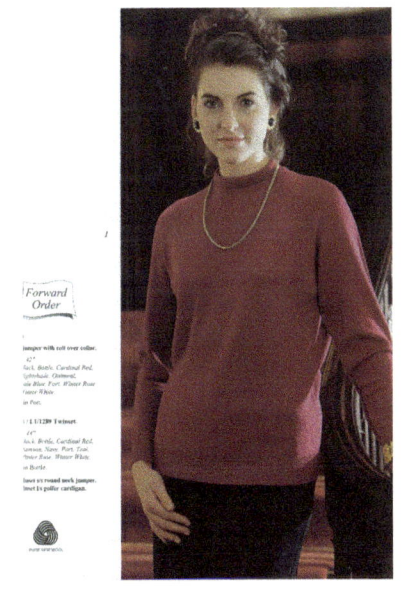

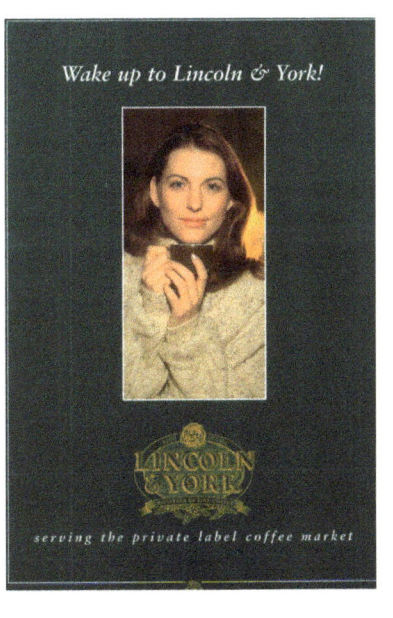

Jeanne modelling a knitting pattern.

Jeanne looking all cosy for Lincoln + York Coffee Makers.

Thursday 10th

We start work on a sofa commercial at 9.15 and we have not been given a finish time as it's a case of you can't go until it's finished. Thankfully it's local and there are a few models on the job so we have a good time. We have to do our own make up and hair plus take a good selection of smart casual. I hate this brief as it could mean anything!!!!

Friday 11th

I have a photoshoot in stevenage. It's only a couple of hours but worth while doing as my petrol is paid. Plus it's for a well known store so I may get some good pictures for my portfolio. (It was for bewise but they have long gone.)

Saturday 12th

I am store walking for country casuals in Birmingham. I love working for these as I get the chance to look at all the store and get paid for it. I have to go and walk round the whole store holding a plaque with the company name on and go throughout the restaurant stopping at the tables chatting to the customers and telling them what deals the brand has on - 25% off or whatever they may have been doing. They normally have drinks and nibbles for people to enjoy whilst browsing the range. (This was very popular in the 70's. Country Casuals always had a very good day with sales when we did this sort of promotion.)

I look through my diary and realise I still have 4 full days straight photographic jobs and a fashion show after, before I have a day off. phew !!!!! But I wouldn't change it for the world. xxx

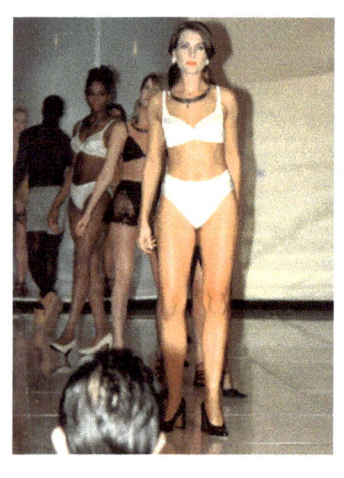

Jeanne modelling lingerie, check out those abs!!

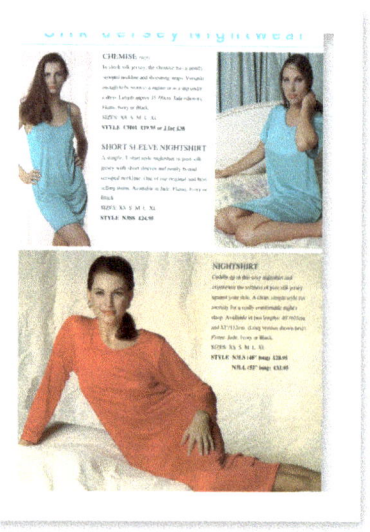

Jeanne modelling Silk Jersey Nightwear – 'Lady in Red'!

Jeanne's Modelling Diary

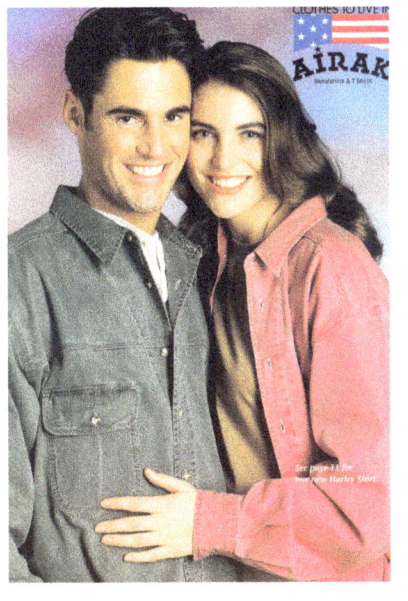

Jeanne modelling for Airak.

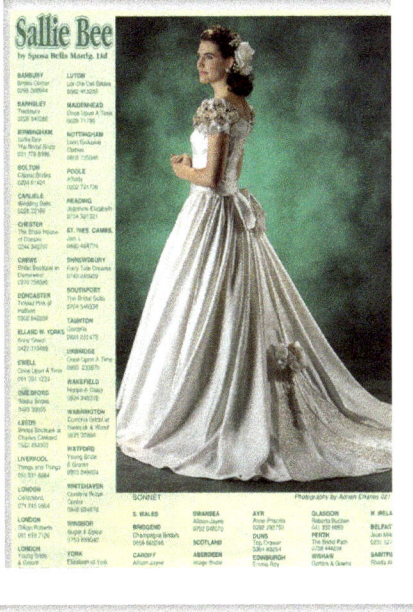

Jeanne modelling for Sallie Bee Bridal.

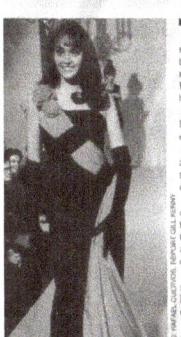
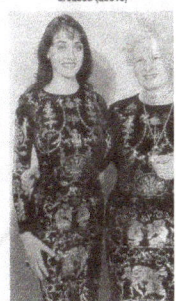

Tiffany featured in Hello! Magazine with Vivienne Westwood.

TIFFANY'S MODELLING DIARY

This is Tiffany's model work diary for one week in 1995.

Sunday:
I'm working outside doing data capture for Marlboro Cigarettes at the British Grand Prix. It is so hot and managed to get fabulous sun burnt T-Shirt marks and I'm doing a photo shoot tomorrow for Berketex Brides.

Monday:
Doing a full day photographic at a studio in Birmingham for Berketex Brides with some fab girlies. I'm being made up by my favourite make up artist too! Bit of a problem - they can't tone down my sunburn from yesterday. Oh dear, client not happy and have called my agency. I'm not going to be on the front cover of the brochure now!! We stood so still like robots all day, I'm fed up of being seen and not heard.

Tuesday:
Casting in London today for hair work with well known celebrity hairdressers. Arrived on time to find at least 60 beautiful girls waiting to be seen so just turned around, headed for the exit and went shopping instead. I get so cross with myself for having zero self confidence.

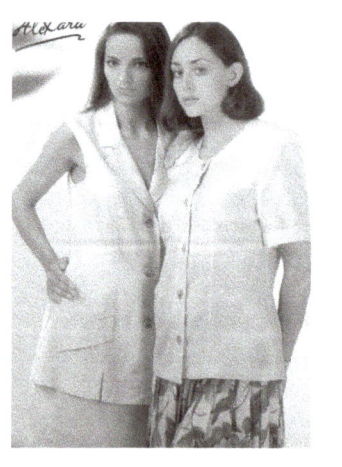

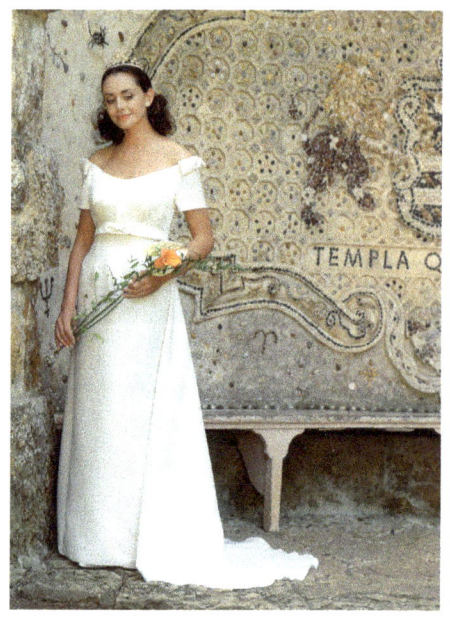

Tiffany modelling clothes- check out the floral skirt! Right: Tiffany modelling for Berketex Brides.

Tiffany's Modelling Diary

Wednesday:
Doing an unpaid photoshoot for Umberto Giannini. He is entering Avante Garde Hairdresser of the Year. Had a great team of experts doing my hair and spraying me silver all over! Ahh I hope I can get this off I've got a lingerie fashion show tomorrow!! Had such a laugh today but finished at 2am what a long day.

Thursday:
Fashion show job in Leicester for students end of year work. It's 7.30am I'm tired and on my way, still got silver bits on some areas of my body. It was a fab day though lots of fun and their families and friends loved the show, the lingerie was amazing! It's 10pm and on my way home.

Friday:
Got a letter from Northampton University today saying I have got a place at their Fashion design course and I start in September yeahhh!!!! Casting in the morning for a Trevor Sorbie Hair road show in Germany, Norway and France and I got it!!

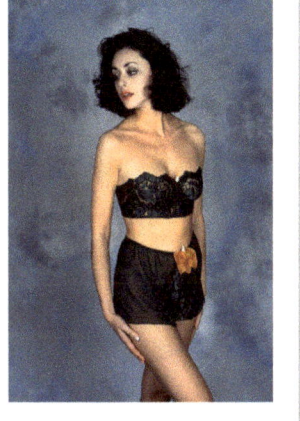
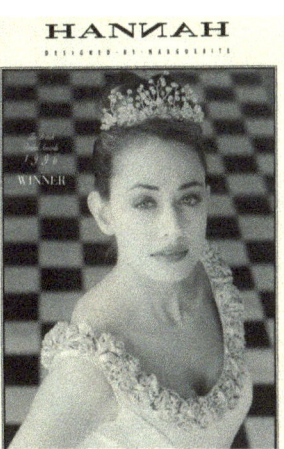

*Left to right: Tiffany modelling for Boots.
Tiffany modelling a student's underwear design...beautiful!
Tiffany modelling Alan Hannah bridal wear.*

Do You Wannabe a Model?

Another Casting today for Harrogate lingerie stand work, the lingerie fitted me well as they needed a girl with a natural size 32 D bust and an 8-10 figure. I was the first to be told to go home so my usual insecure self assumed I hadn't got the job but I did!! I am so pleased as its £200 per day.

Saturday:
Paying for a head shot test shoot with Simon Donnelly, I'm lacking a good Black and White head shot for my portfolio and he is one of my Favourite photographers. I worked with him after I won Face of the Midlands beauty competition.

Sunday:
Full day photographic with Boots in Nottingham for one of their in house leaflets. Boots is closed today hence why we are able to do the shoot. Worked with a gorgeous guy and had such a laugh together, shame I'm not single! We got time and a half too as it was a Sunday, really chuffed!! Need more of these days.

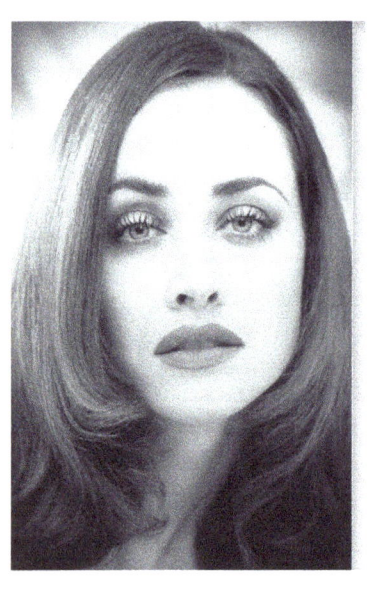

Tiffany's favourite head shot taken by Simon Donelley.

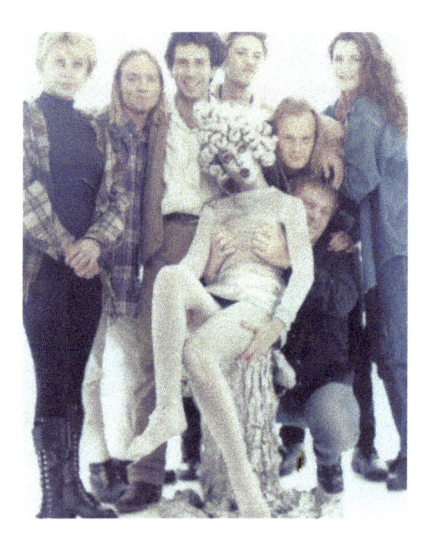

Tiffany modelling for Umberto Giannini.

OUR FINAL WORDS!

We both hope that you have enjoyed our model book. We have written it with the intention of steering potential models in the right direction, to get into the modelling industry and also specifically to help and educate our Wannabe Workshop attendees.

We are unable to guarantee that you will make it as 'Britain's next top model' but we are able to help give you the right knowledge required to get into the modelling industry.

The modelling industry can be fickle and unpredictable so we recommend that you grab any opportunity that comes your way and enjoy the experiences.

Sometimes you may not have good experiences, where for weeks you are not working, or you may be rejected at every casting that you attend, but we both say: "Don't take it personally, keep strong and keep trying." After all, it can be character building!

Through determination and not giving up, we both succeeded in our modelling careers. We believe that it can be the best industry to work in and that's why we are both still involved in it.

We wish you lots of luck and hope you have a very fulfilling career.

Jeanne Frith x
Tiffany Stanford. x

ACKNOWLEDGEMENTS

We would like to thank Mark Webb from Into Print for all your patience and hard work, Helen Mikolajczyk for all your help with ideas and adding all your expert writing magic to our book and to our husbands Ross Williams and Tim Gunner for all your love and support, we love you!

www.ingramcontent.com/pod-product-compliance
Lightning Source LLC
LaVergne TN
LVHW010317070426
835507LV00026B/3429